DOUGHNUTS AND TEMPLES

What is a doughnut?

The Oxford English Reference Dictionary: n. (US donut) **1** a small fried cake of sweetened dough, usu. in the shape of a ball or ring.

What is a temple?

The Oxford English Reference Dictionary: n. **1** a building devoted to the worship, or regarded as the dwelling place, of a god or gods or other objects of religious reverence. **5** a place in which God is regarded as residing, esp. a Christian's person or body.

Holy Bible, New International Version, 1 Cor. 3 verse 16: 'Don't you know that you yourselves are God's temple and that God's Spirit lives in you?'

What's the connection?

A doughnut is made of approximately one-third sugar (including white flour which quickly breaks down into glucose) and one-sixth fat (which, by being cooked at high temperatures, has produced dangerous molecules called free radicals). The average Westerner is reckoned to eat his own body-weight in sugar every year. In addition, as much as 40% of his diet is fat. Yet sugar and poor-grade fats are known to play a part in many serious health conditions, including the three major killers—cancer, heart disease and diabetes, problems which are virtually unknown in underdeveloped countries. Even in Britain as recently as the 1930s, heart attacks were so rare that doctors found them difficult to diagnose.

So, if our bodies are God's temple, what are we doing to them by bringing offerings of junk food—sugar, chemical additives and fats—instead of nutritious, wholesome fare? How much longer can Christians get away with an irresponsible attitude to what they put into their bodies? Doughnuts are clearly just one type of food with very real health risks. It isn't a sin to eat them. Provided we have been born again of the Spirit of God and given our lives to Jesus Christ, we shall still go to heaven when we die, even if we're fond of eating doughnuts; we are just likely to get there sooner. The point is that Christian liberty includes the freedom to make wise choices.

Expanding on her series of columns in *Wholeness* magazine, Nutritionist Erica White explains how the food we eat can cause many common health problems such as fatigue, migraines, high blood pressure, allergies, depression, etc. She suggests that, if we do not have the fullness of life which Jesus promised (*John 10 verse 10*), maybe our 'sweet tooth' is to blame—and the fact that we give it a higher place of worship in the temple than we give to the Holy Spirit.

Is there still one area in the life of many Christians which is not given over to God, an area of self-gratification (or even lust) which means that they eat the things they most desire, even at the expense of their health and an otherwise total commitment to pleasing God? Surely God would rather we co-operate with him for our health than keep running to him for healing?

1 Corinthians 3 verse 17: 'If anyone destroys God's temple, God will destroy him; for God's temple is sacred, and you are that temple.' Are you in danger of destroying your temple?

The underlying challenge in this book is set in the context of the author's own spiritual journey which led her eventually from sickness into health. As the Lord revealed more of himself to her, she came to understand that he wanted her to be well but that he also wanted her to take greater responsibility for the health of her body. Having learned the lesson, at the age of fifty-three she started a three-year training to become a Nutrition Consultant. Erica White is a mother, grandmother and wife. She worships at the Elim Christian Centre in Leigh-on-Sea, Essex, where her husband Robin is an elder.

Doughnuts and Temples

*Be Nice to the Body
God Gave You!*

Erica White

WHITE PUBLICATIONS
Westcliff-on-Sea

First published by Monarch Books 2000
This edition published by White Publications 2004

White Publications, 2 Electric Avenue
Westcliff-on-Sea, Essex, SS0 9NQ, England.

ISBN 0 95214 652 5

Book design and production for the publisher by
Bookprint Creative Services, P.O. Box 827, BN21 3YJ England.
Printed in Great Britain.

DEDICATION

This book is dedicated to all those Christians whose work for the Lord has been disrupted or even cut short by a physical or emotional inability to cope—and to all those for whom this is likely to be the case at some time in the future—simply because they have not been aware that their 'machinery' has been running on low-grade fuel. It comes with a message of encouragement that, by co-operating with God in learning to take greater responsibility for the health of our bodies, the situation in very many cases may be reversed, allowing us as Christians to experience the life in all its fullness which Jesus promised.

'Dear friend, I am praying that all is well with you and that your body is as healthy as I know your soul is' (3 John:2, *Living Bible*).

ACKNOWLEDGMENTS

I learned most of the nutritional information contained in this book at the Institute for Optimum Nutrition in London, and I particularly thank its founder, Patrick Holford, for being a source of great encouragement while he was my tutor, and in the years since. Material used in several of the appendices is largely based upon ION factsheets but with additions by me. I am indebted to Dr Michael Nightingale, a Christian doctor with a keen interest in nutrition, for taking the time to read the manuscript and discuss its content with me, in some places offering encouragement and in others a healthy challenge!

Names of people in this book are either used with their permission or else have been changed to protect their privacy.

The author stresses that readers should seek medical help and diagnosis before attempting self-help treatment for any of the health problems discussed in this book. In addition, this book is written in general terms and no responsibility can be accepted for individual situations where self-help is attempted without appropriate professional guidance.

CONTENTS

FOREWORD

A minister was approached and asked if he would like to take part in a joint venture by local churches. His reply was, 'Oh no, you can count me out. I retire in two years' time and I'm keeping my head down till then.' It is fairly obvious that this sad man was suffering from burnout—exhaustion which had affected him in his body, mind and spirit.

Presumably there had been a time when, as a young Christian, he had heard and responded to the call of God with spiritual fervour, mental zeal and physical vigour. Where had they gone? Surely it is not God's will that, at some stage in our lives, we should pull down the shutters and call it a day? Does there really need to come a time when we have to stop serving God because we are too old, too ill or just plain too tired? At what age do we start to think that we must leave it all to others? Sixty? Fifty? Forty?

Medical progress has led to an increase in life expectancy, but it seems to have done little to improve the *quality* of our lives. Many of us have to curtail our activities as middle-age approaches due to arthritic joints or a general feeling of 'running-down'. Worse still, there is a tremendous increase in premature death by heart attack, which was virtually unknown just sixty years ago. Asthma and eczema have increased six-fold since the 1950s and 150,000 people at any one time in Britain alone are suffering from Chronic Fatigue Syndrome. A third of these are children, so the problems are not confined to mid-life or old age.

There are many causes, including pollution, stress, lifestyle and adulterated food—but a body which is optimally nourished is so much better able to cope that it does not have to succumb to these negative factors. So nutrition is the key, especially when we consider that our modern-day diet is the root cause of most heart attacks, inflammatory conditions, hormonal problems, bowel conditions and weakened immunity.

The idea for this book developed from an invitation to write a regular column on nutrition and health in *Wholeness* magazine. Those articles form the skeleton of Part 2 of this book. In Part 1, I have described incidents of God's work in my life, showing how, little by little, he brought healing to my body and at the same time taught me many things, both physical and spiritual, which eventually led to the work which I now do as a Nutrition Consultant. I believe that my story will testify to God's patience, wisdom and love, and I pray that it will encourage you in your own situation.

However, it is one thing to read how the body is damaged by ignorant or irresponsible eating habits; it is quite another to do something about it to improve your own condition. The book therefore ends with a challenge.

So, be warned—but be well!

Erica White, January 2000

INTRODUCTION

Once upon a time, a long time ago, there was a little girl who was nicknamed Tuppy. She was the only child of loving parents yet, almost from the day she was born, she was never really well. Constant ear-aches, tummy upsets and colds led to her being a nervous child, often away from school, and her otherwise happy teenage years were marred by frequent illness. By the time she was in her twenties and married, she experienced frequent bouts of many different types of '-itis'—sinusitis, fibrositis, cystitis, gastritis, labyrinthitis and more.

The first year she was married, Tuppy experienced a sudden traumatic event; she found she could hardly move her arms and legs or even feel them. Urgent medical tests revealed no apparent cause, but the condition persisted for many months until eventually and inexplicably it went away, just as it had come. It became clear that it had been some type of allergy, a sort of hayfever affecting her whole body which lasted throughout spring and summer, because it returned again the following year, and the next and the next, for many years to come. Antihistamine tablets slightly helped the symptoms, but left her feeling drugged and drowsy.

Tuppy struggled through three pregnancies, suffering

severe sickness and a never-ending barrage of physical problems. Ten days after her third baby was born, she developed excruciating pains which took doctors six months to diagnose as gall-stones. She expected to grow stronger after the operation but instead her health went further downhill, with constant flu-like symptoms. For the next year she spent more time in bed than out of it, depending heavily on her husband, parents and friends to look after the three young children.

Eventually she discovered that all her symptoms of the past year had been caused by another allergy, and this time the culprit was the new domestic gas to which the whole area had just been converted. Immediately, all gas appliances and pipes were removed from the house and Tuppy began to feel better—until she went into another house or building which had the new gas and then all her symptoms would return for several days.

She also found that being exposed to the gas for a whole year had opened the way for other allergies to develop, so now she had severe reactions to several foods and medicines, including antibiotics, also to paint and local anaesthetics, which meant that all her dentistry (and there was a lot) for the next sixteen years had to be endured without injections.

Severe head pains led to the discovery of arthritis in her neck, and many times each year she suffered disabling back pain from a slipped disc, caused initially by falling down some concrete steps onto a station platform. Constant illness, pain, worry and frustration took their toll and, by the time she was thirty-seven, Tuppy was in an anxiety state requiring help from medical tranquillisers. Her life was a mess, physically, mentally—and almost, but not quite—spiritually. When she was a small child she had been taught to pray by her mother. This had opened the door for a relationship with Father God, and now she cried out to him for help.

He answered, first by deepening her relationship with him and increasing her faith, and then by taking her on a journey of discovery which, little by little, led to remarkable changes in her health. It took many years of travelling down a road which was often very bumpy, but Tuppy was carried along by the excitement of each new discovery and by faith that God knew the way he was leading her. She began to realise that very many of the things she learned were to do with nutrition—the effects of food upon her body. At the age of forty, she had to acknowledge that she had never before considered that the food she ate had anything at all to do with her state of constant ill health. On one hand she ate the foods she most enjoyed, and on the other she was always ill.

But Tuppy started to make some discoveries. She found, for instance, that when she stopped drinking coffee, she no longer suffered the miseries of cystitis. When she stopped eating sugary foods, she was no longer exhausted each day by tea-time. When she took certain vitamins, they were more effective at keeping the spring-time allergy at bay than any of the antihistamines which doctors had prescribed, and without the awful drowsiness.

She eventually discovered that many of her remaining problems were due to an overgrowth of a common yeast called *Candida albicans* and, after several years of looking for ways to bring it under control, she realised that she had been led to a nutritional approach which brought eventual victory.

Driving a car had always been exhausting for her. Twenty miles each way was the most she had ever managed but, at the age of fifty-two, Tuppy responded to unusual circumstances by driving several hundred miles in just a few days. She felt well all the time—and loved every minute! Something had changed. A new life had begun.

Perhaps you have guessed that Tuppy is my own nickname, invented by my father and kept up by family and childhood friends throughout my life. In these few paragraphs I have touched on just a fraction of the illness through which I have had to struggle, but God had a purpose in it all.

At the age of fifty-three, just three months after my memorable drive to Wales, I began a course of study to become a Nutrition Consultant. Eleven years later, with three years of training and thousands of consultations behind me, this book is now written as a testimony to God's love and mercy, as an encouragement and a teaching aid—and also as a challenge. I pray that God will open the eyes and ears of your heart and mind to see and hear—and to respond.

Part 1

God at Work

*My health fails; my spirits droop, yet God remains! He is the
strength of my heart; he is mine for ever! . . .
As for me, I get as close to him as I can! I have chosen him
and I will tell everyone about the wonderful ways he rescues
me*

(Psalm 73:26,28, *Living Bible*).

CHAPTER 1

'We have not even heard that there is a Holy Spirit'
(Acts 19:2).

In spite of ongoing health problems of one sort or another, the year 1964 had started well with the birth of our second baby, Emma. She came one cold, January night, with an open fire crackling in the hearth in our bedroom, taking less than two hours to arrive. It was encouraging to know that my body could still do *some* things well!

Her big brother, Toby, had developed projectile vomiting when he was three weeks old; it had been diagnosed as pyloric stenosis and had required urgent surgery on his very little tummy. We had been told that the condition ran in families and, although it was less likely to occur in girls than boys, it was still fairly common so we kept a wary eye on Emma and were very relieved when she showed no signs of it.

When the baby was five months old, I was advised by a gynaecologist that I needed some surgical repairs. During my stay in hospital, my ever-supportive husband Robin became very ill himself. He had always been fit and suffered little illness, but he had looked increasingly grey, and now he was aching all over and was obviously very tired. We thought he just needed a rest, so as soon as I was out of hospital, he took a holiday from work and we packed the babies with their toys and nappies into our little old car and set off to stay with Robin's parents at their beautiful cottage in Kent. It would be a good break and a chance for us both to recuperate. But Robin became increasingly ill, and my convalescence became a nightmare as his pain grew worse. One day, I realised with horror that he was asleep with his eyes open, evidently unable to close them. When he woke, he was barely able to move.

The doctor ordered immediate hospitalisation, but I urged him to let us drive home to Essex first, where I felt I would be better able to cope. The doctor agreed but contacted our own GP and local hospital, where arrangements were made for an immediate bed. A series of tests was put into motion. We had to wait five days for the results but doctors told me some of the possibilities for which they were looking—possible lead poisoning (Robin worked for a print company), brain tumour, stroke, multiple sclerosis or leprosy! Still weak from my operation, I prayed as never before.

Next day the drains broke under our house, and the stench in every room was indescribable. Not knowing whether my husband would live, let alone be able to work again, I set about finding a builder and the money to pay him. Problems were coming at me from every side. I prayed for strength to cope and for protection from panic and I soon found a helpful and reasonable builder so that the drains were mended and the smell began to subside.

The tests showed that Robin had none of the diseases which his doctors had feared. He had a condition called Guillaine Barré syndrome. The cause was unknown, but it was thought that he might have picked up a virus when swimming in the sea. The paralysis had stopped short of his chest, though an 'iron lung' respirator had been standing ready by his door. With treatment and swimming pool therapy, he slowly recovered movement and lost the pain. After six weeks he was well enough to be allowed home, although for four months he was still collected by ambulance each day to go to the hospital pool and also for occupational therapy to increase the mobility of his fingers. He became expert at origami!

I thanked God for my husband's recovery, but the events of that summer had left me pretty shaky. Robin said later that he never once doubted that he would recover, and he is sure now that the Lord gave him a special gift of faith, although at the time he did not know such things were possible!

With daily hospital visits over, I hoped that life would settle down—but the very next day found me back at the hospital! Baby Emma, now nine months old and crawling, followed me into the garden where I was hanging nappies on the line. Suddenly she was screaming, and as I ran to see what was wrong I saw that her little hand was red with blood. A piece of old metal lying in the garden had sliced off the top of her finger. I have never fainted in my life, but I came very close to it then. I grabbed one of the clean nappies, wrapped it round her arm and rang for an ambulance.

In casualty, I was asked when the baby had last had anything to eat or drink. Apparently the top of her finger was still attached, hanging by a thread, and the doctor wanted to see if he could stitch it back on. Emma had only just had some juice when the accident happened, so the operation had to be delayed by four hours because the general anaesthetic would have been too risky. Eventually, it was over and we returned home with a drowsy baby whose little hand was wrapped in a big ball of bandage.

Ten days later, back at the hospital, the doctor inspected

the finger and said that probably due to the time-lapse the operation had not been successful. The finger tip had withered to a large scab, and I was told that they would need to amputate the finger at the lower knuckle.

I was stunned. This was the left-hand ring finger of my baby girl. How terrible to think that it would be just a stump! I tried to concentrate on what the doctor was saying.

'We can do nothing more today,' he said. 'There is still too much infection present. We will treat it, and then you can bring her back in three days' time for the operation.'

Once again, I prayed harder than ever before. I cried out to God for three days and nights that he would somehow save that little finger, but I really had no faith that he would answer. I was simply desperate.

We returned to the hospital after three days and, as instructed, asked for the doctor by name. Eventually a nurse came to apologise that he had been called away, so we would have to see another doctor. I nodded. What difference could it make?

'What's been happening here?' asked the new doctor, as he unwrapped the ball of bandage.

I explained that I had been instructed to bring the baby on this day in order to have her finger amputated. He looked at the tiny finger and I felt sure his face went pale. He looked angry.

'*What* did you say?' he asked.

I repeated what I had said, thinking he had not heard. There was a moment's pause.

'Nonsense!' said the doctor very loudly. 'You should never have been told that!'

'You mean—you're *not* going to amputate?'

'That is exactly what I mean,' said the doctor. 'This is baby tissue. We will leave it well alone and see what happens.'

I burst into tears while the little hand was being wrapped again in bandages. They were tears of tremendous relief but, more than that, they were tears of immense gratitude, for I knew that God had answered my prayers and had supernaturally intervened in the situation by arranging for the first doctor to be called away. I was absolutely overwhelmed with the realisation that God had answered my prayer.

Eventually, the injury was barely noticeable, and even the nail grew back to cover some of the slight deformity. Hardly anyone notices that Emma has a 'special' finger. And special it is, for she not only plays her flute to the praise and glory of God in worship, but on that finger she wears a wedding ring to show that she is married to a minister of God!

What happened to me as a result of this incident was also very special. I walked home from the hospital with Emma in her buggy, and it was not until I caught sight of someone looking at me strangely that I realised what I was doing. Tears were streaming down my face but I was singing quite loudly. It was a simple song which I sang with the children in Sunday school, where I had recently started to teach:

> Thank you, thank you, Jesus,
> Thank you, thank you, Jesus,
> Thank you, thank you, Jesus, from my heart.

There was no room in my mind for any thought or emotion other than tremendous gratitude to God. He had answered my prayers and, in so doing, had made himself more real to me than ever before. I had one objective as I hurried home. I wanted to put the baby in her cot and be on my own with God. I stood in my bedroom, face turned upward, and found that mere words could not express the depth of gratitude that was pouring from my heart.

As I stood there, I was conscious that something was

flowing down over me, as though I was standing in a soft, warm shower. It came onto my head and flowed all down my body. It flowed and flowed and flowed. It was a physical sensation, and somehow I knew it was God's love. It felt like honey. It poured onto me thickly and slowly and seemed to be sticking to me.

I don't know how long I stood there. It was certainly several minutes, but I didn't want it to stop. When eventually it did, I continued to stand, bathed in love and joy and peace. I wrapped my arms around myself, wanting to hold on to this beautiful feeling.

I decided I would tell no one, not even Robin. How could I possibly describe what had happened, and how could I expect someone else to understand? Robin, with his science degree, would have a very logical explanation; he would no doubt say that I had been through a deeply emotional experience, following a draining and difficult time. But I knew it had been more than that, and I didn't want it to be explained away. What happened had not come from my emotions. It had come from an outside source. I knew it had come from God.

This was in 1964, and I had not come across any teaching about the Holy Spirit. When I read my Bible, I had never noticed that Jesus said to his followers, 'You will be baptised with the Holy Spirit' (Acts 1:5).

It took eight whole years for my understanding to catch up with my experience. When Paul asked the Ephesians if they had received the Holy Spirit when they believed, they replied, 'No, we have not even heard that there is a Holy Spirit' (Acts 19:2). My reply would have been the same.

Meanwhile, my health continued to deteriorate.

CHAPTER 2

'Give me also springs of water' (Judges 1:15).

After a couple of years of hugging my secret to myself, I felt increasingly that I wanted to tell Robin what had happened. When I did, to my delight and amazement, he accepted everything I said and did not attempt to use his scientific mind to analyse it. All I could say was, 'I know it came from God'—and Robin believed me! I didn't realise how much the Lord was already at work in my husband also.

Eight years after my special experience, I was still struggling with constant ill health, including the after-effects of a recent gall-bladder operation and the discovery of an allergy to gas which had kept me virtually bed-bound for a year. The wear and tear of all these problems had led to an anxiety state. In Chapter 7 I will show how the Lord broke through in my life and dealt with both anxiety and depression.

Within a few weeks of that incident, Robin was introduced to the brother of an old friend and he invited us to go to a meeting where Christians would be learning about the Holy Spirit. We didn't know what to expect but we felt it would be right to go. When we got there, we certainly didn't enjoy it! About sixty people were squeezed into a small sitting-room, seated in three rings of chairs, one inside the other. By now we had been regular church-goers for some time, but Anglican worship had not prepared us for such extrovert expressions of 'Amen!' and 'Hallelujah!' all through the prayers. We were *most* uncomfortable. However, the talk was to be given by an Anglican vicar, which was reassuring, and it was a great relief when he began to speak.

He read from Judges 1, where newly-married Achsah was encouraged by her husband to ask her father, Caleb, for springs of water to transform the desert land where they would be living, and he had given her 'the upper and the lower springs'. Our speaker identified the upper springs as being the gifts of the Spirit (as listed in 1 Corinthians 12:8–10) which are showered down upon us, and the lower springs as being the fruit of the Spirit (as listed in Galatians 5:22) which well up within us. We were encouraged to ask our heavenly Father for those springs of water which would turn our own arid existence into abundant and fruitful life. It sounded good to me!

When our new friend had invited us to the meeting, he had also lent us a book called *Nine o'clock in the Morning* by Dennis Bennett. As I read it, I remembered my 'honey' experience of eight years before and I realised that, without my even knowing that such a thing could happen, God had poured out his Holy Spirit on me at that time. This being so, what about the gifts and the fruits that seemed to come as part of the Holy Spirit package—the upper and lower springs? Did I, like Achsah, need to ask for them? How important was it that I should have them? I certainly yearned to be free of my arid existence, to have my desert places watered and refreshed.

I came across Deuteronomy 28:65–67, in the *Jerusalem Bible*, where it says:

Among these nations there will be no repose for you, no rest for the sole of your foot; Yahweh (the Lord) will give you a quaking heart, weary eyes, halting breath. Your life from the outset will be a burden to you; night and day you will go in fear, uncertain of your life. In the morning you will say, 'How I wish it were evening!', and in the evening, 'How I wish it were morning!', such terror will grip your heart, such sights your eyes will see.

I thought, 'But that's exactly how I feel! I'm so ill in the daytime that I can't wait to go to bed, and I'm so ill in the night that I can't wait to get up. These verses describe *me*! Yet, incredibly, it says that God will *give* me these things—a quaking heart, weary eyes, fear and all the rest. Why? Why would God give me these terrible things?'

In order to understand, I knew I needed to go back to the start of the paragraph. It said (verse 63):

For not obeying the voice of Yahweh your God, just as Yahweh took delight in giving you prosperity and increase, so now he will take delight in bringing you ruin and destruction.

'But Lord, *what* am I not obeying? I *want* to obey you! What am I not doing?'

I knew I needed to go back even further to the previous paragraph, and there I read (verse 58):

If you do not keep and observe all the words of this Law that are written in this book . . . Yahweh will strike you down with monstrous plagues, you and your descendants: with plagues grievous and lasting, diseases pernicious and enduring.

'Oh, Lord, this is getting worse! Which words of this Law are you talking about?'

The answer came loud and clear, at the start of a paragraph even further back (verse 47):

For failing to serve Yahweh your God in the joy and happiness that come from an abundance of all things, you will submit to the enemies that Yahweh will send against you.

Wait a minute: 'For failing to serve the Lord your God . . .'

I didn't think I was failing there. I served him at Sunday school, for one thing. Sometimes I had to struggle really hard against my health problems to do it, but I very, very seldom failed to get there. It was extremely hard-going, serving the Lord! I certainly wasn't failing in that one!

'. . . in the joy and happiness . . .'

Joy and happiness? Well, as I just said, it's really hard-going, serving the Lord; it's a struggle. How can we be expected to serve him in joy and happiness?

'. . . that come from an abundance of all things . . .'

An abundance? Of all things? Things perhaps that I didn't have? The upper and lower springs to water the desert? Is that what it meant?

'. . . you will submit to the enemies that Yahweh will send against you.'

I suddenly saw it. I had submitted to these enemies of sickness and pain simply because, although I had been serving the Lord, I had been doing it in my own strength and not in his. I had not taken advantage of the resources that were available to me—'the abundance of all things' which would enable me to serve God in joy and happiness instead of with a struggling mind and body.

Obviously, I needed to repent of self-sufficiency, useless as it was, and ask God for the upper and lower springs so that my life might be watered by the Holy Spirit, and made fruitful and abundant.

'But, Lord, why have I never realised this till now?'

He replied immediately, by showing me Deuteronomy 29:3: 'But until today Yahweh has given you no heart to understand, no eyes to see, no ears to hear.'

Clearly, God was saying that I had been blind and deaf long enough, and he had decided today to open my understanding! For eight years I had been living with the whole power and resources of the Holy Spirit available to me, because God had chosen to fill me with his Holy Spirit. But what difference had it made in those eight years?

I had to say that it had seemed to make no difference at all. My health had deteriorated and our problems had escalated after the birth of our third baby, Hannah, in 1969—and this time the new baby *did* have pyloric stenosis. But now it was obvious that all this time God had been waiting; waiting for me to ask him about the beautiful experience he had let me enjoy as he poured out his love on me. Instead, I had hugged it to myself, afraid to lose even the memory of it. And as just a memory it was pretty useless!

Yet many things had happened in those eight years which, looking back, had the special touch of God upon them. As I taught in Sunday school, my own understanding of the Scriptures grew more clear and many of the children eventually went on to serve God with their lives. Our own children developed a real love for Jesus.

So I realised that the work of the Holy Spirit is never without power, but in my own life and physical suffering it was as though nothing had ever happened. Why? Because I had not taken hold of all that the Holy Spirit had for me, his resources of supernatural gifts and fruit.

It was no excuse to say I hadn't known; I should have asked God much sooner what it was he wanted me to learn. Now I believed he had shown me and, in the spring of 1972, I was going to ask for springs of water, in the form of all the resources which the Holy Spirit might have for me, to come into my hard, arid, desert existence and transform it.

CHAPTER 3

'For the Lord trains the ones that he loves . . . Suffering is part of your training' (Hebrews 12:6–7, *Jerusalem Bible*).

It seemed that the Holy Spirit was already giving me a new awareness as I read the Bible and, in the Acts of the Apostles, I noticed that the disciples were always keen to make sure that new Christians received the Holy Spirit. We are either then told that they received the gift of tongues, or that something happened which could be seen or heard by other people, which might well have included speaking in tongues. Simon the magician (Acts 8:9–24) was so impressed that he wanted to buy the power to do it himself. At any rate, the gift of tongues seemed to be important—and available to all those early believers.

In 1972, I knew no one with the gift of tongues but I could see no reason why it should not be just as available to Christians today as it was back in the first century AD. After all, I now knew that I had been filled with the Spirit just like the early Christians, so why shouldn't I be able to receive the gift of tongues like them? I wanted to show God that I meant business.

'Right, Lord. Here I am. I believe you are telling me to take hold of the gift of tongues. If it was part of the package for New Testament believers, there seems no reason why it shouldn't be part of the package for me, too.'

What would happen now?

As I wondered, I realised that for quite some time, several months possibly, a few foreign-sounding words had kept coming into my mind. I hadn't taken too much notice of them; sometimes they were there, and sometimes not. At this moment, they were very much in mind. I decided to speak them out loud. They were definitely foreign words. They made me think of Eastern Europe. I wondered if any more words would come, but I felt it wouldn't happen if I just sat with my mouth open and waited. So I started making sounds and slowly put them together—more words were being formed! All at once, the sounds started to flow. I spoke word after word, quickly and easily. They formed obvious sentences and there was expression in my voice. It really did sound like a foreign language! On and on I spoke, until I thought to look at the time and found that forty-five minutes had passed!

My spirit sang as I realised that God had given me a new language in which I could talk to him! I could express all my love and gratitude, just as I had wanted to do eight years earlier when my prayer that Emma's finger should be saved had been so magnificently answered. Now I had words to do it!

Suddenly, the joy vanished. Doubt and anxiety took over. My mind told me that I had obviously made it all up. It just sounded like someone pretending to speak a foreign language. But, I argued, it seemed strange that I hadn't been able to do it before. Then came the thought that, even worse than me making them up, perhaps the words had come from the devil. How would I know? Perhaps it would be safer not to use them again.

'Oh, Lord, I need to know! If these words are a gift from you, I want to receive them. But if they have just come from my mind, or worse still from the enemy, then I want to drop them like a hot brick! I need to know, but who can I ask? I don't know anyone who could help me. Lord, perhaps it's not right to ask for a sign, but please could you let me know if these words are really from you?'

I had an idea. The reason I was having this long uninterrupted time with God was that Robin had come home from work with a throat infection and very high temperature. He had gone straight to bed and was so feverish that I had decided to sleep downstairs, in order to get some rest and be able to cope in the morning. Once the children were in bed, I was alone and able to spend this extended time with the Lord. I decided to ask God that, if the words were indeed the gift of tongues from him, he would show me by making Robin well enough to go to work in the morning. There seemed little chance of this happening, so I put the whole thing out of my mind and settled down to sleep on the sofa.

Early next morning I was woken by Robin coming downstairs. He looked bright and fresh and was dressed for work. I was amazed.

'Why are you up so early? Surely it isn't time to get up yet?'

I rubbed my eyes and saw that it was very early indeed.

'Well, there's a lot to do today,' said Robin. 'I thought I'd go in an hour earlier than usual.'

With that, he grabbed some breakfast, kissed me goodbye, and went. He had seemed totally well!

As the children got ready for school, there was no time to think about the implications of what had just happened.

Then soon after they had gone, while I was still in my dressing-gown, the doorbell rang. It was ten minutes to nine. On the doorstep stood a smartly-dressed lady, an acquaintance from church.

'May I come in?' she asked. 'And would you please pray for me?'

Nothing like this had ever happened before but, hiding my surprise, I invited her in, glancing round at the untidy room with the ashes still in the fireplace and hoping she wouldn't notice my rather old dressing-gown!

Rosemary had come straight to my house from the school, where she had just left her children. Standing in the playground, waiting for the bell, she had overheard my name being mentioned by a group of young mothers, all from our church. They were discussing a suggestion I had made that some of us should get together to pray for another young mother in the church who was dying of cancer. Sunday by Sunday, I had heard prayers for her 'comfort and upholding', but no one ever actually prayed for her to be healed. I found myself feeling angry about this and hoped that others might feel the same. If I were that young woman, I felt sure I would want people to ask God to heal me! However, my friends had been rather taken aback at the suggestion, and were discussing it in the playground.

But Rosemary had pricked up her ears. She was coping with some very big problems in her own life and she had thought, 'If someone believes that even cancer can be healed through prayer, perhaps they might also believe that God could solve my problems.' So she had come straight from school on the spur of the moment to ask me to pray with her. As she talked, I could 'hear' my new language running through my head, as though my spirit was talking to God while I listened to Rosemary with my mind. I had prayed aloud with others very little, but I found that I could pray easily in response to her request, and I also found myself encouraging her to believe that God would provide the answers to her problems.

That day, four more ladies rang the doorbell and asked if I would pray for them or listen to their problems. (In between, I had managed to get dressed and clear the ashes!) They were all quite different situations but I found each time that I had a certainty about what God wanted me to say. It was a most unusual day, but from then on these events became normal. God had given me the gift of tongues, and he also graciously gave me the sign I had asked for in healing Robin overnight. He then underlined the sign again and again all through that first day and it was evident that, in giving me the gift of tongues, he wanted me to realise that I was now equipped by the Holy Spirit to do a whole new work, a work based on a new but very strong belief that God's desire was to sort out the problems in people's lives. My role was to encourage their faith for this to happen.

Our children grew up in an atmosphere where almost daily they saw sad ladies come into the house but go out with radiant smiles because God had blessed them and renewed their faith. In blessing others, God was blessing our family also. Robin saw and understood what was happening, but it was another two years before the Lord worked in his own life so that he, too, knew the fullness of the Spirit and was led to a complete change of career.

Once, in the early days, the devil tempted me again to doubt that my gift of tongues was from God. But, as I got up one morning, my eyes fell on a passage in my Bible which was open on my bedside table. It was a paragraph set clearly on its own. It said:

For my part, this is my covenant with them, says Yahweh. My
spirit with which I endowed you, and my words that I have put
in your mouth, will not disappear from your mouth, nor from
the mouths of your children, nor from the mouths of your children's children, for ever and ever, says Yahweh

(Isaiah 59:21, *Jerusalem Bible*).

I received that word from God for myself, my children and
my grandchildren yet to come. As a result, all three children
were filled with the Spirit as teenagers and it is a tremendous
joy to see *their* children now growing up in strong Christian
homes, each of them already with a strong and glowing faith
in Jesus.

On that day in 1972, when Robin was amazingly healed of
a throat infection and five ladies came to my door, I knew I
had at last learned what God had been waiting patiently to
teach me. I had discovered the supernatural gifts of the Spirit
as listed in 1 Corinthians 12:1–11, and I had stepped out in
faith to use them. As I spent time with each of the visitors, I
was given words of knowledge and words of wisdom to
speak into their situations; each time, God made it very clear
what he wanted me to do and say.

Little did I know that many years later God would give me
an additional role. The more time I spent in talking and
praying with an ever-growing number of people, the more I
was struck by the fact that quite often their problems had
been brought about by their own irresponsibility. I knew that
God was always willing to forgive and ready to move in on a
situation to heal it and transform it, but I was increasingly
convinced that he would prefer his children to live and act
responsibly so that we did not have to keep running to him
for help.

So when he began to teach me to take responsibility for the
health of my body through making wiser choices about what

I put into it, I knew that he was speaking not only to me but to countless others of my Christian brothers and sisters. I realised that I was to be given the role of raising their awareness about the harm they were doing to themselves, and to show them how to change their eating habits of a lifetime in order to bring healing to their bodies and an increase in strength and vigour. Meanwhile, before I could embark on this mission, I still had a lot to learn myself!

One day, I was struck by some words in Hebrews 12:6–7 (*Jerusalem Bible*), where it says that suffering is part of our training. I could see why the Lord had needed to train me and the means he had used to do it—and I earnestly believed that the time had come when I could say, 'Lord, your word tells us that you use suffering as part of our training. I believe you have allowed me to experience illness so that I would stop trying to be self-sufficient and so that I would learn about the power of your Holy Spirit which is available to me, as a Christian. And I believe that I have now learned this lesson so that, by faith, I may ask you to bring to an end this part of my training, to lift the suffering. So, Lord, would you please now heal me?'

CHAPTER 4

'See, I have delivered Jericho into your hands'
(Joshua 6:2).

I tried to think of someone who might believe in God's healing power and whom I could ask to pray for me. In 1972, I hadn't even heard of churches where healing services were held. Once more, I had to turn to the Lord and ask him for someone to talk to.

I remembered the meeting where we had learned about the upper and lower springs. During that evening I had heard the name of a local Baptist minister whom I had actually met at local Sunday school training days. I was surprised that these 'strange' people knew him. Did he perhaps understand about the Holy Spirit? I decided to contact him and find out if he had any thoughts on healing.

I rang him and told him that I had been filled with the Spirit and was now seeking God's healing for my body. I apologised for troubling him since I was not a member of his flock, but he said he would be happy to come and see me. Later, as I told him all that had happened, he nodded with understanding, and I felt as though God was picking me up and cradling me. It was amazing that I had found someone who understood what I was talking about!

Eventually he said, 'I need to pray about it. I'm still pretty new to all this. I need to be quite certain that God wants me to pray for your healing.'

A week later, he rang and asked, 'When can I come and pray with you?'

He came one Tuesday afternoon in May. He put his hand on my head as I sat, and prayed a simple, believing prayer that I would be healed. I felt an unbelievable peace, both in and around me.

I became aware that the minister was quietly letting himself out of the house, but I just sat and drank in the peace. After a while, I blinked my eyes and picked up the Bible, lying open beside me. It opened at Deuteronomy, and I read: 'Yahweh will keep all sickness far from you; he will not afflict you with those evil plagues of Egypt which you have known' (Deuteronomy 7:15, *Jerusalem Bible*).

The impact of the words, and the timing, was unbelievable. I had just, for the first time in my life, received prayer for healing, and the very first words I read came in the form of a promise that God would keep all sickness far from me. I read on, and 'received' the rest of the passage:

You may say in your heart, 'These nations outnumber me; how shall I be able to dispossess them?' Do not be afraid of them: remember how Yahweh your God dealt with Pharaoh and all Egypt, the great ordeals your own eyes have seen, the signs and wonders, the mighty hand and outstretched arm with which Yahweh your God has brought you out. So will Yahweh your God deal with all the peoples whom you fear to face. And what is more, Yahweh your God will send hornets to destroy those who remain and hide from you. Do not be afraid of them for Yahweh your God is among you, a God who is great and terrible. Little by little Yahweh your God will destroy these nations

before you; you will not be able to make an end of them at once,
or the wild beasts would grow too many for you. But Yahweh
your God will deliver them over to you and will harass them until
they are destroyed. He will deliver their kings into your hands
and you will blot out their names from under heaven; none shall
withstand you, until you have destroyed them all.

(Deuteronomy 7:17–24, *Jerusalem Bible*).

It is extraordinary how quickly our minds jump from spiritual realities to practical problems. I immediately found
myself wondering what I should do about the medicine I was
taking. Should I stop the tablets as an act of faith? Should I
just assume that I was now healed and didn't need them? In
fact, I had asked the minister this question before he prayed
for me, and his wise reply was that this decision could only
be made between God and me.

At the time I was taking antihistamine tablets, on prescription from the doctor. The spring-time allergy had been really
severe and, of course, I still came into contact with gas in
various places. If I took an antihistamine every twelve hours,
it certainly kept the symptoms at bay to a large extent—not
that my doctor believed it was possible to be allergic to gas!

As I wondered what to do, I glanced back down at
Deuteronomy 7. The first two verses said,

When Yahweh your God has led you into the land you are entering to make your own, many nations will fall before you: Hittites,
Girgashites . . . seven nations greater and stronger than yourselves. Yahweh your God will deliver them over to you and you
will conquer them. You must lay them under ban. You must
make no covenant with them nor show them any pity.

(Deuteronomy 7:1–2, *Jerusalem Bible*).

Once again, the Bible seemed to speak directly into my situation. I felt as though I had been making a covenant, an

agreement, with the allergies by taking antihistamines. Was the Lord telling me to stop taking them? I believed he was. I missed out the evening tablet.

As the evening wore on, I began to feel ill. The symptoms got worse and worse. My head ached and swam, my limbs ached and grew heavy, my stomach was increasingly 'wobbly'.

'Lord,' I said, 'I'm prepared to be obedient in order to receive my healing, and I really believe you have told me to stop taking those tablets. But how long shall I have to feel as ill as this?'

As I dragged myself up the stairs to bed, I found myself thinking about the children of Israel as they attacked the walls of Jericho. I remembered the story (in Joshua 6) of how God had told Joshua to instruct the Israelites to march around the walls of the city. They had to do it for six days and then, on the seventh day, they had to march round seven times, with the priests blowing their trumpets and the soldiers shouting a mighty war-cry. God promised that if they would fight this battle by following his instructions, and not by looking to their own strength and reasoning, the walls of Jericho would collapse and the Israelites would be able to capture the city with incredible ease.

I had no idea why Jericho had come into my mind. It was a long time since I had read the story, yet somehow I felt I could identify with the Israelites as they marched around the walls. They were probably dressed for battle, feeling very hot and suffering with bad headaches. They were almost certainly feeling pretty foolish. These men were used to fighting battles, not just walking round city walls! And the inhabitants of Jericho must have been laughing their heads off. What on earth did these stupid Israelites think they were doing?

I had to admit that I felt pretty foolish, too. If anyone knew how ill I was feeling, they would say, 'Why on earth don't you take your tablets?'

All this went through my mind as I slowly climbed the stairs. Before I reached the top, I knew what God was saying. He was telling me to be obedient for seven days, and then the walls of this enemy city would come crashing down. Seven days. Seven days of feeling like this? 'Yes, Lord, if that's what you're telling me. I believe that if I am obedient for seven days and don't make an agreement with the enemy symptoms by taking tablets during that time, after seven days I shall have won the battle, and I shall have won it *your* way!'

I felt terrible for those seven days, but I was so certain that God had spoken that I even told the children and said, 'Please be good and helpful for the next week because I am feeling particularly poorly, but God is going to make me well at the end of it.' If there had been any doubt in my mind at all, I would not have dared to say this, for fear of shattering the growing faith of our three young children. But I was sure.

The Lord gave me his word that I would have sufficient strength to obey him. I read Deuteronomy 30:11–14 (*Jerusalem Bible*), where it says:

> For this Law that I enjoin on you today is not beyond your strength or beyond your reach. It is not in heaven, so that you need to wonder, 'Who will go up to heaven for us and bring it down to us, so that we may hear it and keep it?' Nor is it beyond the seas, so that you need to wonder, 'Who will cross the seas for us and bring it back to us, so that we may hear it and keep it?' No, the Word is very near to you, it is in your mouth and in your heart for your observance.

Robin did his utmost to help me through the week. As he set off in the mornings, he would remind me of the Israelites setting out again to march round Jericho, and say, 'Keep blowing your trumpet!'

One week later we were in a park. It was a fine May evening and we had taken the children out for a little while before bedtime. Robin suddenly looked at me and said, 'Do you realise what you're doing?'

I stopped to consider. 'What?' I asked.

'You're playing ball,' he said.

It was true. For the first time in a very long while, I was playing ball with my family. For many years, I had just sat on a bench and watched. Now I was well enough to play, and I hadn't even realised.

The walls of Jericho had fallen, and I was feeling well.

CHAPTER 5

*'But if your heart turns away and you are not obedient,
and if you are drawn away to bow down to other gods
and worship them, I declare to you this day that you
will certainly be destroyed. You will not live long in the
land you are crossing the Jordan to enter and possess'*
(Deuteronomy 30:17).

At first I felt so well that I didn't stop to wonder about
exactly what had been healed! However, although it soon
became clear that I had not been healed of everything, there
was no doubt at all that my allergic reaction to gas had completely disappeared.

I began to find that I could visit my friends or my parents, in
houses where there was gas, and not be ill. This was certainly
not due to mind over matter, because I was still really scared of
gas. As soon as I went anywhere, I would quickly glance round
to see if there was gas, and panic if I saw a gas fire. But in fact
it never made me ill again. I found I could stay overnight in
houses with gas, and gradually the dread of it began to subside,
dread which had built up through countless horrendous reactions. In fact, we later restored gas central heating and open gas
fires to our home and have had them now for several years.

I have since learned that domestic gas is about the seventh most common allergen, and at one time in Chicago a similar new gas caused an epidemic of sickness, yet in England in the 1970s no doctor would believe me. The Lord knew, however, and he lifted me out of a situation which could not be helped in any other way.

I soon discovered that many problems still remained, and at first these were a puzzle to me. Why had God given me a gift of supernatural healing, but only dealt with one of my problems?

What followed over the following months and years was a growing adventure of discovery, and I realised that God evidently intended me to experience his healing power in many different forms, the first being his direct, supernatural intervention through prayer. I then went on to experience surgery for a prolapsed bladder which had unknowingly been responsible for constant reinfections. Osteopathy followed, and through it I was healed of devastating head pains caused by an unsuspected arthritic neck. And increasingly I learned of ways in which various foods were causing ill health while others could help my body to function more efficiently.

Slowly, I was being restored to health. But just as it had said in Deuteronomy 7, God did not allow me to overcome my enemies all at once; it was happening 'little by little'. I still had frequent sickness and pain due to various different causes. There was obviously more I had to learn. As I pressed forward, determined to find more answers, I found myself going down a few blind alleys which would have led me into dangerous territory had God not kept his hand upon me.

At the time of the head pains, which were later discovered to be caused by an osteo-arthritic neck, someone suggested acupuncture. We heard of an established clinic about twenty miles away, and I went twice for treatment. Twice was more than enough! Each time I returned home feeling absolutely dreadful; obviously, this was not the intended result so something must be very wrong. I couldn't face the third appointment. I didn't understand for some years why this should have happened when so many other people claim to have received such help from acupuncture.

In 1985, I thought I had found an answer to many of my problems in homeopathy. The benefits appeared to be twofold; first, that my continuing sinus problems seemed much better, especially the intermittent attacks of vertigo, but, even more importantly, the treatment was guaranteed to stop allergic reactions to anaesthetics. This had become an important consideration because, in a few months' time, I would be having another 'gynae' operation. It was thirteen years since I had last received a general anaesthetic and, during those years, I had developed major reactions to local anaesthetics, so no one now could be sure how I might react to a general one. Not surprisingly, I was pretty scared.

A few weeks before I was due to go into hospital, we went for the very first time to Faith Camp, to receive teaching and ministry from Colin Urquhart and Bob Gordon. This was our first time at a big Christian camp. On the Monday morning, we went to a seminar called 'Roadblocks to Progress', and one of the blocks mentioned was alternative medicine, including homeopathy. I had already come across a disapproving attitude towards it in some Christians, which I thought was quite ridiculous. After all, I was feeling so much better. Now I had to listen to this man going on about it! I began to lose patience with him. As far as I could see, homeopathy was a perfectly natural and safe alternative to the drugs used in orthodox medicine. Why, some very famous people, including members of the Royal Family, have homeopathic doctors! What did this man think he knew?

'Homeopathy,' said the speaker at Faith Camp, 'is from the pit.' And then, just as if he could hear me arguing with him, he went on, 'And if you don't believe me, I'll give you the name of someone else you can talk to about it.'

Robin and I looked at each other. We knew we had to follow this through. I was angry, and I was also frightened, but I would not now be able to rest until I had found out as much as I could about homeopathy.

The Christian man to whom we went to speak had practised homeopathy for twenty years, believing it to be a perfectly valid and helpful form of medicine, until the Lord had shown him in various ways that it had its roots in the occult. I couldn't believe this, but I listened to his explanation. He said that no medical or scientific approach has been able to explain the healing power of homeopathy, so where does its power come from? For power it undoubtedly has! Most people believe that homeopathy was originated by a Dr Hahnemann in the early nineteenth century, but in fact Hahnemann had based his theories on the writings of Paracelsus, an alchemist and astrologer who lived in the fifteenth century and who believed that the stars and occult forces governed sickness and who also considered himself to be greater than God!

This all came as quite a shock, but I still felt pretty sceptical. Our new friend told us of several experiences which had increased his understanding that, as a practising homeopath, he was moving in the realms of the occult until, finally, he knew he had to renounce it.

As I listened, I tried to consider what it meant for me.

And then he said, 'You know, I have found that whenever a Christian has been treated by homeopathic remedies, it has dulled their spiritual sensitivity.'

A bell rang in my head. Was this what it was all about? For the past thirteen years I had been involved in counselling and praying with people. I was not in the business of just giving good advice, but of needing to hear what God wanted me to do and say in each situation. I had to make use of the gifts of the Spirit, which are really the tools available to us for doing God's work. I needed to have discernment of evil, words of knowledge, words of wisdom, and so on. After all, if somebody said they were depressed, I needed to know the root cause of that depression. It could be physical, possibly due to a hormonal imbalance or a viral infection; it could be a mental or emotional reaction to circumstances; or it could be due entirely to a spiritual demonic attack. If I was going to be used in helping that person, I needed to know what I was dealing with. I needed to be able to hear from God. And that took spiritual sensitivity.

My mind raced on. If the enemy was interested in trying to stop the work I was doing for God, he would probably first try physical attack. He certainly liked using that one on me! But increasingly he had found that attacking me physically had not had the desired effect. The prayer and the counselling continued even if I was stuck in a chair for six months, as had once been the case. He obviously needed to try another tactic.

And now I knew, with utter certainty, that the tactic he had used was to get me to rely on homeopathic remedies in order that my spiritual sensitivity would be dulled. I knew then that I had to renounce homeopathy, and repent to God of my involvement with it, regardless of my fear of what might happen with the anaesthetic.

I prayed a prayer of repentance, asking the Lord to forgive me and wash me clean of all the effects of homeopathy. Over the next two days, all the symptoms which had been helped by the homeopathic remedies came flooding back—intense sinus headache, giddiness, aching, general weakness.

I was determined not to let these symptoms hold me back from entering into all that was happening at the camp, including the early morning praise time, and with a tremendous effort I got out of bed to be there and I sang and praised the Lord even though my head was crashing and reeling. I believed that the way was now clear for the Lord to come in and heal me—there was nothing now to block it. At the next evening's meeting, ill as I was, I responded in faith with Robin when people were asked to go forward for prayer if they knew that God was asking them to serve him in some full-time capacity. With all our hearts, that is what we both wanted, but it could only be possible if God gave me health; he was asking me to step out in faith that he would indeed complete the healing in my body which he had so marvellously begun.

The following evening, the power of God suddenly came down upon me where I stood, in the midst of several thousand people, and I fell onto the row of chairs behind me. I was aware of all that was happening, but I felt as though I was resting in the presence of God. The next night we went to Ishmael's Praise Party, and I danced and sang with as much joy as Ishmael himself; I was no longer giddy and my headache had completely gone!

A few weeks later I had the operation. The anaesthetist was very attentive to my history of allergy, and he tried small amounts of different substances to see how I would react. I remember losing consciousness, saying, 'Yes, thank you, this one's fine . . .' and awaking quite safely some time later.

I hadn't needed homeopathy to protect me from the anaesthetic, nor did I need any form of therapy which, because of its origins and underlying beliefs, was not pleasing to God. I learned later that acupuncture is rooted in Chinese spiritual philosophy, which is very far removed from Christianity.

Roy Livesey, in his book *More Understanding Alternative Medicine*, says that when Satan is invited in, however unknowingly, he will leave something behind that was not bargained for. It was indeed unknowingly that I had given the enemy opportunities to gain entry into my life through homeopathy and acupuncture, and once more I had been quite unaware of the devil's tactics.

But I had given my life to Jesus and, protected as I was by him, the enemy did not gain the stronghold in my life for which he had plotted and schemed. Paul once wrote, 'Let your armour be the Lord Jesus Christ!' (Romans 13:14). Being clothed and covered and surrounded by Jesus is certainly the safest place to be!

CHAPTER 6

'For I know the plans I have for you,' declares the Lord,
'plans to prosper you and not to harm you, plans to give
you hope and a future' (Jeremiah 29:11).

One of the biggest steps on my journey to health came
through learning about a minute microbe which lives inside
each one of us but which very readily overgrows and
migrates throughout the body, causing umpteen problems,
given the right circumstances. It is a yeast called *Candida
albicans*, and you will find a whole chapter of this book
devoted to it!

The discovery of candida, and what to do about it, eventually led in 1988 to such an improvement in my health that
people noticed the difference and began to ask whether I
could help them with their own health problems. I was very
aware of my inadequate knowledge and wondered whether
there might be some sort of training I could do. I had never
heard of a nutritionist at the time.

One day a friend lent me a copy of a health magazine in
which was a notice about a diploma course being run by the
Institute for Optimum Nutrition in London for people
wishing to become Nutrition Consultants. Was this what I

should do? Would they accept a grandma as a student? It was pretty expensive; could we afford it?

We thought and prayed, and the idea of training just wouldn't leave me. I made some enquiries which led to an interview, after which I was offered a place for September, in just two months' time! What had I done? What sort of studying would be involved? I had left school at seventeen with a handful of O-levels followed by an excellent secretarial course, but that was the extent of my academic career and I had not studied for thirty-six years!

It was necessary for me to do a basic science foundation course before I could begin, and Robin's years as a science teacher were a tremendous blessing to me. I enrolled as a satellite student, which meant I could listen to the lectures on tapes at home and send in my homework assignments, but I would also have to attend several weekends in each term for seminars and workshops.

Having tussled with the foundation course, I looked at the timetable of work ahead and was utterly overwhelmed. Biochemistry, physiology, nutrition, a research project to set up—the syllabus and the reading list were literally heavy!

We turned our smallest bedroom into a study with some second-hand furniture and, as I studied, more and more people were telephoning for advice. I told them the little I knew—and, to my amazement, many became well! Soon we had to buy an answerphone to switch on at mealtimes. I produced sheets of information and found I was being asked to send them all over the country. With all this happening, my studying was done mostly late at night—yet my stamina continued to hold out. I was aware that a lot of people had begun to rely on me, but I knew with complete certainty that I, in turn, could rely on God. Sometimes I had an opportunity to tell people how God had healed me, and sometimes they would ask me to pray with them.

Homework marks were coming in, and they were encouraging. Perhaps I could do it, after all! My research project required volunteers suffering from eating disorders and, as I advised them on diet and supplied them with amino acid supplements, I saw some amazing results. One lady had been secretly bulimic for thirty years, since the age of twelve, and she also suffered multiple joint pain. After just ten weeks, she was completely free of both!

I graduated with distinction at the end of two years, only to return three years later for another year of study which had just been added to upgrade the course. In addition, I kept up with continuous post-graduate training including learning about some medicinal uses of herbs to help alleviate symptoms while nutritional therapy gets to the root of the problem.

I became so busy that we decided it was right for Robin to give up teaching, as a step of faith, in order to take over the administration from me. Within a short space of time, we needed to employ more helpers until eventually we were a team of nine. We made a habit, very early on, of praying together once a week for those clients who particularly seemed to need it or who specifically asked for prayer.

I was invited back to give lectures at the Institute where I had trained, and increasingly invitations came in to speak to groups and churches, both locally and further afield, from Inverness to the United Arab Emirates! I also found time to write, publishing books on candida and ME, and receiving other commissions. The number of consultations, both with people coming to see me and those whom I advised by post, came close to a thousand in each year.

At the time of life when I should have been retired, I found myself busier and healthier than ever before. The Lord had repaid me for the years that the locusts had eaten (Joel 2:25)! Having recovered the health which had been stolen from me, I now had the privilege of helping others to regain theirs.

There are many chronic health problems for which the medical profession acknowledges that it has no answers apart from helping to relieve pain or depression. Very often in these situations, it is the nutritional status which is at fault. A consultant neurologist began to refer many people to me, all of them suffering from chronic fatigue, because he saw those of his patients who had also received nutritional advice very often showed that enormous improvements could be achieved simply by making changes in diet and taking a tailor-made programme of vitamins and minerals. My favourite comment came from a Yorkshire doctor who said, 'This lassie knows what she's on about'!

It is obvious, when you think about it, that since our body's machinery is dependent on food for its fuel, it will work better when it is well nourished. The problem is, of course, that each of us has completely different inherited strengths and weaknesses, as well as different medical histories, lifestyles and eating habits, so each one of us needs a tailor-made programme to repair nutritional deficiencies and imbalances in the body's cells and tissues. It is what is known as 'biochemical individuality', and it requires a well-trained technique on the part of a nutritionist, using extremely detailed questionnaires, to assess individual requirements and formulate a suitable programme to encourage each of the body's systems to work with greatest efficiency.

And making these detailed assessments and recommendations is what I found myself doing, for countless hours in every week, as more and more people were helped and word of mouth began to snowball.

It is amazing to think that the Lord had this plan in mind through all the years when he was patiently waiting for me to discover what he wanted me to learn, both in the spiritual and the physical realms. My one regret is that it took me so long to ask him to show me, but as I look back (as I occasionally do when I can find the time to stop!), the sense of joy and fulfilment is tremendous when I compare my previous arid existence with the fullness of life which now is mine, just as Jesus promised to each one of us (John 10:10).

My hope is that the chapters which follow will throw some light on stubborn health problems which may be afflicting you or someone you love. I have given simple advice on each topic which at least should set you in the right direction, and throughout you will read more testimonies—sometimes mine, sometimes those of clients. I hope these true stories will help you to share my belief that God, omnipotent as he is, actually longs for us to co-operate with him for our health and our healing, and I hope then that you will be able to say 'Amen' to the challenge with which this book ends!

Part 2

Nutrition as God Intended

Then God said, 'I give you every seed-bearing plant on the
face of the whole earth and every tree that has fruit with seed
in it. They will be yours for food'

(Genesis 1:29).

Every living and crawling thing shall provide food for you, no
less than the foliage of plants

(Genesis 9:3, *Jerusalem Bible*).

CHAPTER 7

MOODY BLUES—ANXIETY AND DEPRESSION

'. . . the darkness in this world' (Ephesians 6:12, *Jerusalem Bible*).

By the age of thirty-seven, the wear and tear of constant ill health had left its mark. It seemed that I was never without an infection of some type, and there were frequent bouts of severe pain from my problem back, teeth, sinuses and muscles. Added to this were the debilitating complications caused by various allergies. Trying to bring up a family of three small children involved a daily battle with my body to find the strength. I was exhausted, and exhaustion led to an anxiety state, for which I was prescribed tranquillisers.

Throughout these years, Robin and I had maintained a sort of link with the church, which had increased since we had moved to Leigh-on-Sea nine years before. In spite of my poor health, I somehow never thought of myself as ailing, and I undertook various commitments with Sunday school and women's meetings. However, the struggle to keep them up just added to my overall exhaustion. One Sunday we were together in church as a family, and during a time of prayer, I found myself shaking uncontrollably with anxiety, even though I was already taking prescribed tranquillisers. I had no idea what had caused this but it suddenly struck me that, as a Christian, I should be experiencing joy and peace during this time of prayer in the Lord's house. So what had gone wrong?

I decided the time had come to sort it out with God himself. I needed a time when I could be on my own with him, and Monday morning would be the first opportunity, with even Hannah, our youngest, out of the house at nursery school. But first I had to get through Sunday, and so Robin took the children out while I just lay on the sofa and shook.

On Monday morning at nine o'clock I was ready for my appointment with God. I didn't know what to do or expect, so I just sat and poured out everything to him, crying and speaking aloud, with tears streaming down my face, until all my troubles were laid at his feet. Only then did I stop. What now? What could I expect to happen?

Within moments, a very clear thought came into my mind: 'What you need is the armour of God.' The armour of God—I could remember teaching about it in Sunday school. I had drawn a visual aid of the helmet, the shield and all the other pieces. I flicked through my copy of the *Jerusalem Bible* till I found the description of the armour of God in Ephesians 6. As I read it I knew straight away that every word was being spoken by God directly to me.

Verse 10: Finally, grow strong in the Lord, with the strength of his power.

I certainly needed to do that. My own strength had completely failed me.

Verse 11: Put God's armour on so as to be able to resist the devil's tactics.

The devil? Did he really exist? I'd never given him a second thought. Yet the Bible was saying that he not only exists but that he uses tactics against us which we need to resist. What an amazing thought!

> Verse 12: For it is not against human enemies that we have to struggle but against the Sovereignties and the Powers who originate the darkness in this world, the spiritual army of evil in the heavens.

To my mind, there was nothing darker in this world than depression. I used to think that if I wasn't depressed I would be able to cope with almost anything, but I had been under a dark cloud for so long that even a splinter in my finger seemed too much to cope with. And where did the Bible say depression came from? From the 'Sovereignties and Powers who originate the darkness in this world, the spiritual army of evil in the heavens'. An army? Warfare? In heaven?

> Verse 13: That is why you must rely on God's armour, or you will not be able to put up any resistance when the worst happens, or have enough resources to hold your ground.

Wasn't that exactly what I was afraid of? That if something really bad happened within the family, for instance, I would never be able to cope, because at the moment I could barely even cope with normal everyday existence. And the Bible was saying that I was absolutely right to be afraid; it actually confirmed that I would *not* be able to put up any resistance when the worst happened, or have enough resources to hold my ground—*unless* . . . unless I learned to rely on the armour which God had provided.

I have since compared this translation with others many

times, and in no other version is the imperative tense written so strongly: you *must* rely on God's armour if you want to stand against the devil's schemes and tactics.

How did God know that this was exactly what I needed to hear? Well, hadn't I just told him—poured out to him all my fears? And within minutes he had answered me at my deepest point of need, speaking straight into my anxiety.

I began to see that the root of it was a lack of assurance that I would ever again be well; I didn't know if God would heal me, or even if he wanted to. And now, for the first time, I began to see that my suffering was not from God but from the devil, and, with that realisation, a ray of light which was almost physical broke through into my mind. If my suffering actually came from the enemy, there was hope that God's purpose for my life might be something quite different. Since God is stronger than the devil, perhaps I could now begin to believe that he really wanted to heal me; perhaps now I could really expect to be healed. Could I? Dare I hope for that? Why else was God speaking to me in this way?

Verse 14: So stand your ground, with truth buckled round your waist, and integrity for a breastplate.

What did 'truth' mean to me at that moment? I felt as though God was telling me to hold on to the truth of all that he had so far shown me about my situation; many medical tests had looked for nasty underlying diseases, and they had all come back with negative results. I felt I was being told to hold on to that, not to let my imagination run away with me by suggesting that maybe I had leukaemia, for instance, and that really I was dying!

God had allowed me to know certain facts and I felt that

in due course much more would come clear. Meanwhile, I was to hold on to the truth of what I had been told so far. That would certainly help to strengthen me against uncontrolled anxiety.

What about 'integrity'? I learned later that most other versions use the word 'righteousness', which would have led my thinking in other directions, but here I was being told to use 'integrity for a breastplate'. I felt I was being shown that I should have integrity, honesty, in my relationships, in my dealings with God and with people. It occurred to me that quite often friends would say, 'Oh, you poor thing, are you ill again?' And I would reply, 'Well, yes, I am,'—and I would immediately feel a 'poor thing' and my spirit would crash down into a black pit.

I knew that in future my reply would have to change. 'Are you ill again?' 'Yes, but I believe that God is healing me.' What a statement of faith that would be! Could I be that bold? I believed I could. Speaking out my faith would be acting with integrity on what God had said to me. And instead of being pulled down by well-meaning friends, I would be built up by speaking out my faith in God's desire and ability to heal me. I could see how it would happen, and in that way integrity would certainly be a valuable piece of armour.

Some more recent translations of the Bible have interpreted 'righteousness' or 'integrity' as 'God's approval'. What a mind-blowing thought that is! And yet of course it is quite possible for us to have God's approval if we have given our lives to him, because now we are living in Jesus who has covered our sins by dying for us.

Verse 15: Wearing for shoes on your feet the eagerness to spread the gospel of peace.

Well, if what I was discovering now was the gospel of peace to replace the lies of anxiety, I would certainly want to share it with other needy people. But before I could spread it, I would need to get hold of it for myself. What a motivation! What a splendid piece of armour—eagerness on my feet!

> Verse 16: And always carrying the shield of faith so that you can use it to put out the burning arrows of the evil one.

I had never thought of anxiety attacks as being burning arrows, but that's exactly what they were like; panic that pierced right through to the inner being. But if I had the shield of faith in position, those arrows would bounce off it and land useless on the ground. The devil might aim his arrows at me, but they would not be able to penetrate and I would not be harmed. This was getting pretty exciting!

> Verse 17: And then you must accept salvation from God to be your helmet.

That word 'must' again! But how exactly do you 'accept salvation'? My understanding of salvation was that it had taken place two thousand years ago, when Jesus died on the cross so that I might be saved. I realised it also meant that, at some time in the future, when I died, I could be certain of going to heaven, because I loved Jesus and knew him to be the Son of God—which in fact I had never doubted. It struck me that these amazing truths, based on the past and the future, should have such a tremendous impact on the present that I would be continuously, overwhelmingly full of joy and peace and gratitude!

And the Bible didn't say you should *try* to live in this state

of accepting salvation; it said, 'You *must* . . .'! If I didn't, if
I lived in gloom and despair instead of joy and praise, this
particular piece of armour, the helmet, would be useless—
and the enemy would have a straight line of entry into my
head, into my thoughts and imagination.

Verse 17: —and receive the word of God from the Spirit to use
as a sword.

That is exactly what I was doing! For the very first time I
had recognised my enemy and I had been given a sword with
which to fight him—a word from God in my heart and mind
which had pointed me to his written word, the Bible. I was
no longer just trying to defend my ground; I was fighting
back.

Verse 18: Pray all the time, asking for what you need, praying in
the Spirit on every possible occasion.

So it isn't wrong to pray for yourself, as Christians often
seem to think. The Bible actually says that we should ask for
what we need. How tremendously reassuring! But what about
'praying in the Spirit'? I didn't know what that meant, but
perhaps it included pouring your heart out to God and receiving his reply, as I had just experienced. Had that been the
Spirit of God communicating with mine? I was intrigued and
on fire to understand more.

The effect on me of these discoveries was gradual but
steady. Each morning I read the passage in Ephesians before
I dared get out of bed and face the day—and each day I experienced less and less anxiety. I began to hear the Lord speaking to me in other passages, too, and my times with the Bible
became an adventure. After a couple of months I was able to

stop taking tranquillisers and I have since been grateful to the medical knowledge that enabled me to have a brief period of mild sedation, because without it I believe my mind was too agitated to have been able to hear what God was trying to say to me.

Soon I came across the passage in Hebrews which I have described in Chapter 3:

> The Lord trains the ones that he loves and he punishes all those that he acknowledges as his sons. Suffering is part of your training; God is treating you as his sons
>
> (Hebrews 12:6–7, *Jerusalem Bible*).

I thought I knew a lot about suffering, but I had no idea that it could be used by God to train us. I cried out to him to show me what he wanted me to learn, so that the training, the suffering, could be lifted. Looking back, I am amazed that I had never thought of this before; it could have saved me years of trouble. Now that it occurred to me to ask God what he was wanting me to learn, he lost no time in giving me a very clear answer. He wanted me to learn about the Holy Spirit and, more than that, to understand and recognise that I had already been filled with the Holy Spirit eight long years before.

So the root of my anxiety state had been spiritual, but with hindsight it is obvious that the enemy was taking advantage, not only of my lack of armour but also of my weakened physical state due to the fact that I was suffering from various biochemical conditions—low blood sugar, a body full of candida toxins and several unpleasant allergies.

These are just some of the physical conditions which can give rise to anxiety and depression. There are many others, and some are covered in this book. They include adrenal fatigue, hormone imbalance, toxicity (including the effects of prescription medicines), underactive thyroid, nutritional deficiencies, high or low histamine status, a virus or yeast infection and chronic fatigue syndrome (ME).

It is true that the darkness in this world is originated by 'the spiritual army of evil in the heavens', but if we take responsibility for our health in order to overcome such physical conditions, we deprive the enemy of an easy foothold into our lives.

Of course, not all attacks of anxiety or depression are due to a physical situation. Anxiety can come with the threat of redundancy or when facing an exam or an operation. Depression can come with bereavement or failure to get a job. Most of us have experienced times in our lives when we have grappled with circumstances and wondered where God has gone.

There may be situations when the anxiety or depression is without any apparent physical or circumstantial cause; this is where the enemy has caused a spiritual oppression. The situation needs to be recognised and dealt with strongly, calmly and prayerfully in the name of Jesus. 'I have given you authority . . . to overcome all the power of the enemy,' he said (Luke 10:19). We need to take hold of that authority and use it.

If you are living with anxiety or depression, and if there is any suspicion at all that there may be a physical cause—even if any physical symptoms you have seem totally unconnected—you need to pray for wisdom, and maybe God will tell you to seek help from a nutritionist!

I have purposely chosen to make this chapter the first in the section on overcoming health problems. It forms an introduction to the chapters which are to follow by putting our physical symptoms and conditions into the context of spiritual warfare. But we have a loving Father who wants to bless us with peace, joy and health. The third letter of John, written to his friend Gaius, starts with a prayer that 'you may enjoy good health and that all may go well with you, even as your soul is getting along well' (3 John:2).

If God allows us to be ill, it is so that we will draw close to him, learn how to receive his love, grow in faith—and take up the armour he has provided for us so that we may be able to stand against the enemy. There is so much our Father wants to teach us, including how to be well!

Having discovered just how much the enemy had been running rings round me, the rest of my education was just about to begin.

Wise Words
'Cast all your anxiety on him because he cares for you'
(1 Peter 5:7).

For Action
- **Carefully read through Ephesians 6:1–10,** asking God to help you apply his word to your own situation.
- **Carefully read through other chapters in this book** to see if they throw any light upon a physical explanation for your anxiety or depression. Ask God to shine his light onto any physical aspect which requires attention. Consider in particular the possibility of low blood sugar (Chapter 8), allergy (Chapter 9), candida (Chapter 10), chronic fatigue (Chapter 11), hormonal imbalance (Chapter 16), toxicity (Chapter 17) and adrenal exhaustion (Chapter 18). An imbalance in nutritional status alone, which is relevant to all these conditions, is sufficient to cause severe disruption to the emotions.

- If none of these conditions seem to apply in your case, **recognise the situation as warfare, put on your armour and start fighting back with the sword of the Spirit!**

CHAPTER 8

THE UPS AND DOWNS OF LIFE— BLOOD SUGAR AND ENERGY LEVELS

'They will run and not grow weary, they will walk and not be faint' (Isaiah 40:31).

In my early forties, I experienced a regular state of collapse which happened every day at tea-time. Quite suddenly, I would become totally drained, exhausted and giddy. I would have to sit in a chair, absolutely still, unable even to turn my eyes sideways for fear of 'keeling over'. I was far too weak to talk. I just sat there feeling ill, old and grey, not even able to bother about my children.

My doctor could offer no explanation. As far as he was concerned, this was just another one of the strange sufferings of this poor woman whose file grew fatter and fatter.

But Robin discovered something which helped. As soon as I collapsed, he would quickly prepare a plate of food and put it on my lap. I ate it slowly, bite by bite, not moving my head or my eyes, until gradually the food would restore some life and strength to my body and, after a while, I would be able to move and would even cope with putting the children to bed and reading them their stories.

A friend lent me a book entitled *Let's Get Well* by an American nutritionist called Adelle Davis. I read it with real amazement. Adelle described many symptoms and conditions with which I was all too familiar, but she also explained how to tackle them with diet and with vitamins and minerals. Until then I had thought that you just ate what you most enjoyed and your body did its own thing. This was when I first made the connection that food had something to do with my appalling state of ill health.

A whole new way of thinking opened up to me; for the first time in my life I realised that food affects the body. In fact, it is the fuel which makes our machinery work, just like petrol in a car. The fuel I had put into my body for more than thirty years had probably been about the lowest grade imaginable!

From Adelle Davis's description, I was certain that I had a condition called low blood sugar, or hypoglycaemia. Although she went into quite a lot of detail about how to deal with it, I felt I really needed more help. For one thing, I needed to plan a radical change of diet, and I also needed to sort out various vitamins and minerals, including some I had never heard of, so it all seemed quite complicated. Again, I prayed for help—and again the Lord answered, this time by bringing someone all the way across the Atlantic from Boston, Massachusetts!

One Sunday morning I was in church with nine-year-old Hannah. At that time, we normally went to the evening service because the older children preferred it, but Hannah and I went on this particular morning because she wanted to see a friend's baby being christened. We usually sat near the front of the church, but this time we sat near the back, close to the font where the action would be. Everything was different from usual.

A mother and her small girl came and sat in the seats beside us. We had barely started singing the first hymn when the little girl needed the toilet. While they were gone another lady arrived late and slipped into the seat next to mine. I thought it would hardly be welcoming to say she was sitting in someone's place, so when the little girl and her mother returned, we all shuffled up to make room. I later marvelled at how many factors had been carefully arranged so that the visitor should be right next to me.

It soon became clear that she didn't know the order of service or her way through the books so I began to help her and point things out, and we nodded and smiled at each other until we were able to chat at the end, by which time we felt quite like old friends!

Her name was Laura. She had an American accent, although I discovered that she was English by birth but had married an American soldier at the end of the second world war and had lived in Massachusetts ever since. She had returned to England for the sad task of settling her elderly mother into residential care and selling up the family home and contents. She would be in England for a month and would obviously be very lonely, living in a house with grad-ually-decreasing furniture and comforts around her.

I invited her to come to us in the evenings whenever she liked. We became good friends and the Lord, as ever, had it perfectly planned because he had more than one purpose in view. Laura had been seeking to know more about the Holy Spirit and his gifts so I was only too willing to tell her of my own experience and to pray with her. This was obviously one part of God's purpose in bringing us together.

The other part was to answer my prayer for help in over-coming low blood sugar, because it just so happened that Laura had once suffered with hypoglycaemia herself but had been completely cured in an American clinic by following a careful diet and taking a programme of vitamins and minerals. She was able to tell me the information I so much needed and wanted to know, and when she returned to America she sent me several books to help me even further. Among other things, I learned the importance of not eating sugar and of having a protein snack every couple of hours while my blood sugar levels were being regulated. I took specific vitamins and minerals—and soon began to feel very much better indeed!

The Lord had stage-managed a special coming-together of two of his children, normally divided by the Atlantic Ocean, to meet their individual needs. It proved to be another stepping-stone in my understanding that nutrition is important to healing and to health.

Many people who now consult me for nutritional advice speak of a yo-yo effect in their energy levels throughout the day. Remembering my own daily state of collapse, I understand and sympathise only too well. In the morning they find it hard to get going after a restless night, but an early-morning cup of tea or coffee helps them on their way, with perhaps a hurried piece of toast for breakfast. By eleven o'clock their energy is flagging and, like Pooh Bear, they are more than ready for 'a little something'—another cup of coffee and perhaps a biscuit or a doughnut. After that they feel more on top of things and can cope until lunch-time, but by then they certainly need another coffee or perhaps some cola with their white-bread sandwich and chocolate bar.

The afternoon is increasingly difficult as they struggle with headaches and tiredness. Tea and biscuits are essential to get them through the rest of the day. Once home from work, they feel so drained that not even a pizza followed by ice-cream and apple pie from a packet can restore their flagging energy. They then drink several cups of coffee to get them through the evening, which is spent slumped in a chair, sleeping through several TV programmes and eventually stirring just enough to go upstairs to bed. After a restless night, they feel quite unable to start the new day without a cup of tea or coffee to help them force their eyelids open. Sound familiar? This is hypoglycaemia.

Do you suppose this is how life is meant to be lived? Is this what Jesus had in mind when he said, 'I have come that they may have life, and have it to the full' (John 10:10)? In that verse he also speaks of a thief, and we have to admit that it sounds very much as though the robber has managed to steal the gift which Jesus gave. It surely cannot be right!

Let me explain what is happening, and how we give the thief plenty of opportunity to deprive us of an abundant life. Sugar in the blood (glucose) is needed to provide energy to every cell in the body, including the brain, but when sugar levels are low, you are likely to experience any or all of a multitude of symptoms including fatigue or exhaustion, irritability, aggression, nervousness, depression, crying spells, dizziness, fear, anxiety, panic attacks, confusion, forgetfulness, inability to concentrate, insomnia, headaches, palpitations, sweating, fainting, muscle pains, digestive problems, etc. Quite a list! However, the answer to the problem of low blood sugar, surprising as it may seem, is *not* just to eat more sugar!

Imagine a piece of graph paper with a chart drawn across it to indicate levels of sugar in the blood. If you have hypoglycaemia, every time you eat food which has been sweetened with sugar (like biscuits, cakes, puddings, sweets or ice-cream), or something which quickly turns to glucose once digested (like white rice or white flour in bread, pastry, biscuits or cakes), and every time you drink stimulants like tea, coffee, alcohol or cola drinks, the level of glucose in your blood is quickly increased and the line on the graph shoots up to a high point. If it stayed there, you would obviously have high blood sugar, which develops into diabetes, so the body very cleverly does something to avoid this happening. A message is sent to the pancreas to release some insulin, and this makes the sugar levels in your blood drop to a very low point on the graph by encouraging the sugar to be taken up into the cells of your body.

However, the moment when sugar levels in your blood drop to a low point is the moment when you feel your worst, with any or all of the possible symptoms. You might feel dizzy or faint, develop a headache, become irritable or depressed, or have a sudden panic attack, or just feel plain exhausted.

So what do you do? You grab something quickly to give you a 'lift', something which you know from experience will act as a pick-me-up. It might be tea or coffee, a biscuit, a bar of chocolate, a pint of beer or a lady-like sip of sherry—or even a dastardly doughnut!

The symptoms pass; you feel better and able to cope once more, but sadly the new-found energy doesn't last very long. Within a couple of hours you feel just as bad as before—or maybe even worse. This is because the stimulants or the sugar you've just eaten have again increased the level of sugar in your blood to a high point on the graph, so down has gone the message to the pancreas once more, out has come the insulin, and down has plummeted the sugar level in your blood. So what happens next? Out comes the coffee or the sherry or the doughnut, up goes your sugar level—and so the day goes on.

Sugar in the blood gives energy, so energy levels and symptoms of low blood sugar throughout the day swing up and down like a yo-yo, until by evening it is virtually impossible to achieve a balance and you end up totally exhausted. That's exactly what was happening to me every day at tea-time.

More and more sugar or stimulants are needed in order just to keep going, and an addiction to tea, coffee, chocolate, sugar, nicotine or alcohol sets in.

The pancreas starts to over-react and becomes trigger-happy, so the line on the graph goes from high to low to high to low and so on, right across the page. The parts of the body which are trying to control the situation become increasingly exhausted and the situation grows steadily worse. Eventually the pancreas is so exhausted that it stops producing insulin and then there is no way of bringing sugar levels down. Late on-set diabetes has developed. Fortunately, something can be done to prevent this happening.

You need to change the line on the graph from a violent yo-yo effect of peaks and troughs to a gentle, undulating curve of slight ups and downs. You can do this by eating the right sort of foods—those which release small amounts of sugar into your blood quite slowly—and also by eating at frequent intervals so that you 'catch' the falling line on your graph before it drops too low, which is now less likely to happen in any case because of the reduced sugar-intake and consequent reduced output of insulin.

You also need to take some helpful supplements. For instance, Vitamin B3 and the mineral chromium together help the liver to produce an important substance called Glucose Tolerance Factor, which is essential to the control of the body's sugar levels. Vitamin B6, zinc and manganese are also important, and Vitamin B5 and Vitamin C are necessary to support the adrenal glands while things get back to normal—which mercifully they can!

By improving glucose tolerance (in other words, by correcting hypoglycaemia or low blood sugar), you remove a load from the adrenal glands and the pancreas so that they no longer suffer from exhaustion and are able to function efficiently and healthily once more.

An appropriate eating programme involves avoiding sucrose or other added sugars, eating a whole-grain, wholefood diet and also eating little and often. The type of foods chosen should be those which provide energy to the body slowly but surely—good quality proteins like fish, chicken, eggs, natural yoghurt, tofu, beans, lentils and other pulses like chickpeas. In addition, there should be plenty of lightly-steamed or raw vegetables as in salads and also whole grains as in wholemeal bread, wholewheat pasta and wholegrain rice. These are all complex carbohydrates.

Fruit is also a complex carbohydrate but unfortunately it contains fructose which is a natural sugar. Although fructose is absorbed more slowly than sucrose, it still increases the sugar in the blood at some point and should therefore be restricted in the initial stages. Oranges should be completely avoided. Fresh fruit juice of any kind, without the flesh and fibre of the fruit to slow down its absorption, gives a very potent top-up to sugar in the bloodstream and so should also be completely avoided, as should drinks which have been artificially sweetened.

The very best balance of foods in our diet is two-thirds complex carbohydrates to one-third protein. This may be measured by weight or even quite roughly by judging how much would cover the palm of your hand. However approximately estimated, an attempt to follow this guide-line should be made at every single meal and even at every single snack.

In 1995 a book was launched in America called *The Zone*

by Dr Barry Sears (Regan Books). 'The Zone' is the name given to what he describes as the metabolic state in which the body works at peak efficiency. Living in the Zone leads not only to greater energy and physical performance but also to improved mental focus and productivity. So how do we achieve it?

To quote Barry Sears:

> Every time you open your mouth to eat, you're applying for a passport to the Zone. To get that passport, though, you must treat food as if it were a drug. You must eat food in a controlled fashion and in the proper proportions—as if it were an intravenous drip. Reaching the Zone is a matter of dietary technology which is as precise as any computer technology.
>
> The trouble is that most of us are using the wrong rules—eating the wrong foods, or, just as bad, eating the right foods in the wrong proportions. So our access to the Zone is being constantly denied. But follow the rules and your entrance is ensured. It's science. The rewards of increased energy, vitality and performance—in work, in play, in personal relationships—will amaze you.
>
> If this sounds like New Age jargon, it's not. It's the application of twenty-first century biotechnology solutions to a twentieth-century problem—how to increase the efficiency of the human body.

The Zone makes fascinating reading and goes into great detail about how to calculate the actual amounts of protein and complex carbohydrate required according to individual body weight and size and activity levels, but the basis is that you should eat these foods in the right proportions and at the right intervals, ideally spread throughout the day as five light meals rather than three heavy ones. This ties in well with my own advice for correcting low blood sugar.

A Zone-favourable meal should also include a small

amount of fat. Like fibre in wholegrain foods, fat slows down the rate at which carbohydrates enter the bloodstream. However, there are good fats and bad fats. The ones to avoid are saturated animal fats (as in red meat and whole-fat milk and cheese). Good fats suggested by Barry Sears include olive oil (and of course olives themselves), natural peanut butter, avocado, almonds and tahini (made from ground sesame seeds). All these are rich sources of monounsaturated fats. Personally, I would expand the list to include polyunsaturated fats like those found in oily fish, and in sunflower, pumpkin and flax seeds.

We don't need a lot of these beneficial oils, but we do need some. The question is, how much? Just three olives or onethird of a teaspoon of extra-virgin olive oil or half a teaspoon of natural peanut butter is all you need at each snack, with twice as much at a larger meal. It isn't very much, but that small amount is extremely important.

The Zone had not been written when I was sorting out my own blood sugar problems, but with the help of Adelle Davis and my new friend from America, I simply cut out all sugar and refined grains, made sure that I ate frequent portions of protein and complex carbohydrates and swallowed the recommended vitamins and minerals. My blood sugar balance not only improved remarkably at the time but has remained well balanced ever since. My stamina is so constant that from time to time I undertake a three-day fast and hardly notice it! Compared with the appalling energy slumps I experienced as a younger woman, I really can say that I now live life to the full, just as Jesus promised. And so can you.

Please note that fasting, even for spiritual reasons, is quite dangerous if you suffer from hypoglycaemia. You are likely to faint while shopping—or worse, have a black-out while driving the car. Regulating your blood sugar levels means that if the minister/leaders of your church call for a time of prayer and fasting, you will be free to join in to the full and suffer far less than most of your friends.

Wise Words

'Those who hope in the Lord will *renew their strength. They* will *soar on wings like eagles; they* will *run and not grow weary, they* will *walk and not be faint'!* (Isaiah 40:31, my emphases).

For Action

- **Study Appendix A for ways to improve your glucose tolerance,** and determine to put the advice into practice, right down to cutting out sugar, tea, coffee and chocolate!
- **Study Appendix M and determine to improve your eating habits** so that they are more in line with nutrition as God intended.
- **Take regular exercise,** but obviously within your present physical capabilities. You can't beat walking briskly for twenty minutes, at least three times a week.
- **Do all you can to avoid or deal with stress.**
- **Take an appropriate supplement programme** (see Appendix A) to help support and regulate your body's blood sugar control systems.
- **Don't forget to hope in the Lord! He promises to renew your strength.** (See again Isaiah 40:31).

CHAPTER 9

ERRATIC REACTIONS—ALLERGY

'Which of you, if his son asks for bread, will give him a stone? Or if he asks for a fish, will give him a snake?'
(Matthew 7:9–10).

When we were newly married and living in London, Robin invited a friend for dinner. I scoured my new cookbooks and, as it was summer, decided on an exotic salad. I bought lots of colourful things from the market in Portobello Road, and went home to wash and chop and prepare an elegant meal. Within moments of touching a long red pepper, my hands and my face were burning and enormously swollen. I was desperately plunging my hands in cold water, with a wet towel thrown over my head and face, when Robin arrived with our visitor! They rushed me to hospital, where an allergy to chilli peppers was quickly diagnosed. This was my first experience of allergy.

The following March, while shopping in my lunch-break, I felt an odd sensation in my legs. As I tried to walk on, they felt strange—heavy and dragging. My head felt weird as well, as though full of fog. Fighting to keep calm, I went back to work—but my fingers would not type. In a state of panic, I was quickly sent home by taxi with a friend who first called Robin and then rang the doctor. I was taken to a hospital for nervous diseases and prodded and poked by a consultant neurologist and his band of students, but no explanation for my symptoms was found. I was sent home, feeling ill and very frightened. What was wrong with me? Would it get even worse? Was I becoming completely paralysed?

Robin drove me to my parents' house in the country to be looked after, but days became weeks and nothing changed. The aching was intense. My mother massaged my arms and legs, which was comforting but did not really help. Weeks turned into months until, at the end of July, I realised I was feeling better. The aches had subsided, my arms and legs felt normal and my head was clear. Needless to say, this was a tremendous relief, even though there was still no explanation. I put it behind me and got on with my life—but the following March, it happened again.

It didn't take too much detection to realise that, since the symptoms had returned at the same time of year, I must be allergic to some kind of pollen or tree. The doctor prescribed antihistamines which, after an initial few days of making me feel drugged, brought real improvement, and I needed to take them for the next four months. It happened every year for thirteen years; I called it my spring-time allergy, although it lasted well into summer. It was nothing like hay-fever; in fact, it affected almost every part of my body *except* my nose!

In the worst years of my ill health, I developed other allergies. When our youngest baby, Hannah, was born, she developed pyloric stenosis just like her big brother, Toby, and she had to have an operation at just five weeks old—at exactly the same time as I developed excruciating pain which was later found to be caused by gall-stones! It actually took six months for the gall-stones to be diagnosed because my doctor was convinced that I was suffering from post-natal depression. Admittedly, the situation was extremely stressful; the pains I had were unbelievable, and at the same time I was desperately trying to continue to breast-feed a baby who was steadily losing weight because of projectile vomiting, but I knew without doubt that the pain was not just a figment of my mind.

When Hannah was six months old and fully recovered from her operation, I had my gall-bladder removed, complete with stones, and went home to start enjoying life with my three children, but it was not to be. Within weeks I was more ill than ever. I felt severely 'spaced-out', with constant headaches, exhaustion, muscle aches, stomach upsets, palpitations and acute anxiety. It began quite suddenly. Robin was travelling to Italy on a business trip that day, and I couldn't believe I was feeling so ill just because I was slightly nervous that he was going away, yet I presumed this was what it must be.

Somehow I struggled on for a whole year. If I managed to get to the shops at the end of our road, no more than two hundred yards away, I would have to spend the rest of the day on the bed, too weak to do anything else, with palpitations shaking the whole of my body. I had to rely on friends and parents to help with the children, taking them to and from their infant and nursery schools. That year, I spent more time in bed than out of it.

I went away to spend two weeks with an aunt to see if this would help. At first I felt terrible, but by the second week I started to improve. This was tremendously encouraging, yet as soon as I was home the symptoms all returned.

One Sunday afternoon, I was lying in bed feeling definitely more dead than alive. Robin was trying to comfort and support me as well as look after the children. I remember feeling that, in order to stay alive, I had to concentrate hard on something—so we played game after game of 'Battleships' with pencils and paper. Robin had sent for the doctor and eventually an elderly locum arrived.

'Tell me how you feel,' he said.

'I feel as though I'm dying,' was all I could reply.

'Sounds like an allergy,' said the doctor immediately.

He turned back the bed-clothes and pulled up my night-dress to expose my tummy. Using his thumb-nail, he drew lines across my skin. As we watched, the thin scratch marks turned into wide, red weals, which then stayed for a good ten minutes.

'Just as I thought,' said the wise doctor. 'You can play noughts and crosses on an allergy patient!' And he wrote out a prescription for some antihistamine tablets.

Again, once over the initial drowsiness, the tablets certainly helped. But what could possibly be causing such a severe and lengthy reaction? No one seemed particularly bothered or able to find out. It was my mother who eventually came up with an idea.

She suggested that I might be reacting to the new North Sea gas which had been installed in our house the previous year—in fact just two days before Robin flew to Italy and the problems had begun. I have to confess that at first we laughed at my mother's silly idea, but she insisted that her friend had suffered from really severe asthma since the new gas had been installed, and she thought that possibly in some way it might also be affecting me.

Well, anything was worth a try. It was summer so the heaters were all turned off and the only gas being used was for cooking. We decided that for a week I should stay upstairs in the bedroom, not using the kitchen at all and keeping all doors firmly shut. Robin left me with supplies of a vacuum flask and sandwiches each morning, so that I could stay upstairs and out of the kitchen.

By the end of the week's experiment I was definitely feeling better, so we quickly arranged to go all-electric. Not only the gas cooker and heaters were removed, but all the gas pipes from under the house, right out to the pavement.

I was very much better, but we soon made two more discoveries. The first was that when I went anywhere near gas in another house or building, I would experience a return of all the old symptoms and be ill for four or five days. It would happen whether or not I knew there was gas in the building. Sometimes I would become ill and wonder why, but if we retraced my steps of the previous day we would invariably find a gas heater tucked behind a shop counter, or something similar.

The second discovery was that I was now allergic to many other things, presumably because my immune system had been exposed to the gas for so long. In particular, the smell of paint would give me a blazing headache and set off all the old symptoms. The worst problem was finding that I had become allergic to local anaesthetics. The reaction to them was so severe that for the next sixteen years I had all my dentistry without an anaesthetic, including three crowns in one go!

The first of the reactions I have described, to chilli peppers, was a contact reaction; I hadn't even yet got round to eating them! The other two reactions were environmental sensitivities. Over the years, I also discovered that I had some food intolerances.

I once decided to avoid potatoes in order to lose weight. One weekend, Robin and I drove to Hereford for a long weekend to visit Hannah, now grown up and working there as an optometrist. We stopped for lunch at a pretty pub but it had a very limited choice of food. I was already avoiding bread and cheese, having discovered that my body didn't like them (although I did!), and as there were no salads I decided to go for what seemed 'safest'—egg and chips. After just a few mouthfuls, my vision seemed to go foggy. I tried to shake off this odd sensation and continued to eat and chat, happily looking forward to seeing our youngest offspring after quite a long time.

Looking back, I can't think why I ignored the warning signs except that I was really enjoying the egg and chips! But by the time I had finished, the room was in a fog, I was fighting to keep my eye-lids open and I had the beginnings of an almighty headache.

As we continued our journey, all warm feelings of anticipation disappeared. I just felt ill. I also felt incredibly depressed. I looked at a woman on the pavement and wondered if she would die before I did!

The foggy vision, severe headache and black depression completely ruined our weekend away. We stayed in a farmhouse with a four-poster bed and I remember lying in it feeling quite convinced that I was about to die. After a few days, as we returned back home, the symptoms lifted.

There was no doubt at all that potatoes were the culprit. By avoiding them for a while I had unmasked a 'hidden allergy', yet previously I had eaten potatoes—lots of them, all through my life—with no idea that they might be adding to my long list of health problems.

At the time of discovering each of the allergies, it was sufficient relief to find the explanation of the dreadful symptoms and to avoid the offending substances. This was easy with chilli peppers and potatoes, not so easy with gas—and downright impossible with springtime! So little by little, the Lord showed me ways of dealing with the situations.

What is an allergy? It's a term which is used by different people to mean different things. One view is that it should be used only in cases of a severe reaction, leading to anaphylactic shock, to substances like peanuts, lobster or bee-stings, for which some people need urgent hospital treatment to counteract the effects and even save their lives.

More commonly, 'allergy' is used of situations like hay-fever, where pollen leads to a reaction in people who are sensitive to it. A food intolerance is also often called an allergy. Culprit foods can often be difficult to trace, because the reaction might not occur for several hours. I was fortunate in being able to pin-point potatoes so easily because of the immediate reaction they caused. The problem is that the more frequently a culprit food is eaten, the more 'masked' symptoms become, yet the ongoing load on the immune system leads to increasingly chronic ill health.

Allergy is an abnormal reaction to an ordinarily harmless substance which might be inhaled, swallowed, injected or touched. I had all of those!

Many food allergies are due to leaky intestines which allow minute particles of undigested protein to invade the bloodstream; others are due to a lack of digestive enzymes. Hypersensitivity to environmental substances—pollen, dust, gas, animals, fumes—usually happens when the immune system is already overloaded in other ways and starts to shoot off wildly in all directions. An overgrowth of the common yeast, *Candida albicans*, is frequently responsible for both these situations and so needs to be recognised and dealt with first (see Chapter 10).

Allergic symptoms include asthma, eczema, hay-fever, sinusitis, brain-fag, fatigue, migraine, depression, panic, irritability, hyperactivity, hives, inflammation of the joints and muscles, bloating, swelling of the eyes or lips, rashes, constipation, diarrhoea and irritable bowel syndrome. Common culprits include pollen, mould, dust, fur, feathers, stings, perfume, chemicals, medicines and foods, especially wheat and dairy produce. Food allergy is often a cause of obstinate overweight, because fluids are retained to dilute the culprit food and lessen its impact on the immune system. Many people have a hidden sensitivity without having the first idea that this is why they feel unwell or are unable to shift their stubborn excess weight.

Asthma in children is reported to have doubled since the 1970s. Alexander Stalmatski, in his book *Freedom from Asthma* (Kyle Cathie), published in 1997, states that 'Surveys of UK schoolchildren conducted over the last ten years all point to the startling fact that in this country one child in eight now has asthma. There are now some three million asthmatics in the UK. Every week around 40 people die from asthma in this country.' In America, 5,000 people are reported to die of asthma every year, and, in Australia, 'One in four children and one in ten adults are already diagnosed as having the disease. By the year 2020 medical authorities expect that one person in two will have asthma.'

Although allergy may not always be the root cause of asthma, it is certainly one of the major triggers and therefore one of the main reasons why asthma is so much on the increase. What are the reasons for this growth in allergic conditions which indicate that the immunity of this generation has become weaker than ever before?

One factor is that the past fifty years have been the era of antibiotics. Such powerful drugs should enable us to live healthier and stronger lives but instead we seem to develop more and more health problems. Part of the reason for this is that antibiotics encourage an imbalance, or dysbiosis, in the intestines, allowing an overgrowth of unfriendly microbes such as yeasts which cause the gut wall to become leaky. Another factor is that bottle-fed babies do not receive the natural immunity they would derive from the friendly bacteria in breast-milk, and cow's milk in a bottle formula has a very high tendency to cause allergy.

Steroid drugs have become widely used over the past few decades, including cortisone creams and inhalers. It is known that steroids suppress the immune system but it is not generally realised that any form of hormone therapy (and that includes the contraceptive pill) is a form of steroid treatment, so thousands of women and girls are unaware of the fact that day by day they are weakening the strength of their immune systems by taking the Pill or HRT.

Of course, pollution also places a tremendous load on the immune system and, because of the adulterated state of our modern food, the poor old immune system does not even get the nutrients it needs to fight off common, minor bugs, let alone have added strength to deal with pollution and toxins.

Food allergy often 'equals' addiction. If you are unknowingly addicted to a food or drink (possibly tea, coffee, chocolate, alcohol, wheat, dairy produce or potatoes—or almost anything else you can think of!) and if some time has passed since you last ate or drank it, you begin to get withdrawal symptoms. You probably don't recognise it as such; you just feel a bit 'low' or tired or irritable or develop a headache. Because you don't feel too well, you reach for the very thing which experience has taught you will give you a 'lift', just as you do when blood sugar drops. It might be a cup of tea or coffee, a glass of wine or beer, a bar of chocolate or a doughnut—which contains not only sugar and fat but also wheat, one of the most common allergens. You can suspect that you might be addicted to something if you have to acknowledge that you would hate to give it up, and this in turn is a pretty good indication that you are in fact allergic to it, and that the 'lift' it gives is simply fooling you.

So what can be done? Obviously, it helps to pinpoint the culprits and avoid them in order to remove loads from the immune system. At the end of this chapter and in Appendix B you will find advice on how to pinpoint a culprit food. It is important to rid the body of candida overgrowths and take nutritional steps to heal the leaky gut wall. Often, it eventually becomes possible to reintroduce a previous culprit food without problem.

Dealing with candida will not only help to overcome food intolerances but it will also help to reduce inhaled or contact sensitivities. However, it is still essential to strengthen the immune system by eating healthy foods and taking appropriate vitamins and minerals. For instance, through reading *Let's Get Well* by Adelle Davis (Unwin), I discovered that high levels of Vitamins C and B5 worked better than antihistamines, and after that I took them successfully each year throughout the time of my 'spring-time allergy'. Eventually, as I studied nutrition and learned how to take nutritional steps to strengthen my immunity, I found one year that the symptoms did not return.

We also need to be aware that we must fight on the spiritual front, as well as on the physical. Our enemy looks for opportunities to rob us of our health, joy, peace and freedom, so he enables normally harmless substances to poison us by taking advantage of our physical weaknesses. The answer is to rebuild the strength of our bodies by co-operating with God and eating those foods which he originally intended to be fuel for our machinery. If you look at the packets and tins in your kitchen, you will agree that not much of what is listed is food which Jesus would have recognised.

But let us not forget also that if we really are willing to co-operate with God and do whatever he asks of us, he is more than ready to step in and help us, sometimes in quite dramatic ways, just as he freed me from an allergy to gas.

In fact, I barely remember my allergies now. I confess to avoiding chilli peppers and I don't really bother with potatoes, but I have no spring-time problems and I love our open gas fires. Perhaps most of all I rejoice in visiting my dentist because, after sixteen years without, I am able to have a local anaesthetic again! To gain freedom from all these reactions I had to realise that I must stop putting rubbish into my body, because it is God's holy temple. In this way I was able to deprive the enemy of his ability to poison me with food and spring-time blossom!

Our Father does not give us stones instead of bread, or a snake when we have asked for fish. He has provided good things for us to eat. But, given any sort of foothold, the enemy can arrange for food to turn to poison in our bodies— so let's deprive him of those footholds. Let's restore the health of our bodies by co-operating with God in eating the foods which he designed instead of the rubbish designed by humans! If we don't, we ourselves might be held responsible for bringing about our own ill health, for destroying God's temple.

Wise Words

'Don't you know that you yourselves are God's temple and that God's Spirit lives in you? If anyone destroys God's temple, God will destroy him; for God's temple is sacred, and you are that temple' (1 Corinthians 3:16).

For Action

- **If you suspect a food allergy,** decide what you eat or drink most often and avoid it for two weeks to see if you start to feel better.
- **To confirm a food allergy,** after avoiding the food as above, carry out a simple pulse test (see Appendix B).
- **Food should be tested in families,** eg wheat, oats, rye, barley (gluten grains); cow's milk, cheese, yoghurt, butter (dairy produce); potatoes, tomatoes, peppers, aubergines (nightshade family).
- **Try to think if you feel worse in certain environments,** eg where there is mould, or animals, or gas or the smell of glue or paint. If you suspect something, do what you can to avoid it, eg avoid mould by giving away your house-plants; the mould from damp soil in pots in your home becomes airborne and you breathe it in!
- **Change to a wholefood, healthy diet,** free of sugar, junk food, stimulants and chemical additives (see Appendix M).
- **Take a good multivitamin and mineral supplement,** at the very least, to strengthen your immune system. Work out your optimum nutritional requirements. There are books to help, like *The Optimum Nutrition Bible* by Patrick Holford (Piatkus). Or consult a nutritionist for a tailor-made programme.
- **If suffering from hay-fever or asthma,** try taking Vitamin C 1000mg × 3 up to four times daily (stop when it causes diarrhoea) and each time take calcium pantothenate (Vitamin B5) 250mg.
- **Cut down or preferably avoid using bronchodilators** for asthma, rhinitis and sinusitis, and with your doctor's agreement try to avoid steroid inhalers and also steroid creams for eczema; steroids suppress immunity. **Learn about breathing techniques** for alleviating asthma and

sinusitis by reading *Freedom from Asthma* by Alexander Stalmatski (Kyle Cathie).

- **Use an alternative contraceptive to the Pill** and ask your doctor about **stopping HRT**; both of them are steroids and suppress immunity. There are better ways of overcoming menopausal symptoms through nutrition.

- **Food allergies frequently indicate that you have a problem with candida** which has helped to make your intestinal wall become porous—leaky gut syndrome (see Chapter 10). You need to get this under control and then take steps to heal the intestinal lining by taking appropriate nutritional products. It is best to get advice from a nutritionist.

- **Pray that the Holy Spirit will lead you into all truth.** Ours is a very practical God and he is more than willing and able to help you discover and overcome your sensitivities and intolerances.

CHAPTER 10

BEASTLY YEAST—*CANDIDA ALBICANS*

'. . . the owner of the house must go and tell the priest, "I have seen something that looks like mildew in my house"' (Leviticus 14:35).

In 1985, I first heard about yeast infection. I had started ordering vitamins from a company who sometimes enclosed an interesting article. This one described a yeast which normally lives inside each one of us but which, under certain circumstances, increases in number and causes a wide variety of symptoms, both physical and mental. Its name is *Candida albicans*, and the ill health which it causes is called yeast infection, or candidiasis.

The leaflet said that it is difficult to bring candida under control, but that it can be done by keeping to a very special diet, designed to 'starve' the yeast and stop it thriving. It also said that it is necessary to take vitamins and minerals to strengthen immunity and an anti-fungal drug prescribed by your doctor. The symptoms described in the leaflet sounded so much like my own (sinus and nasal problems, bowel problems, headaches, depression, infections of the vagina, kidney and bladder) that I went straight off to discuss it with my doctor. However, he did not agree with the article and refused to prescribe an anti-fungal drug so I decided that I just had to do what I could on my own and work out the special diet. I stuck to it faithfully but, although convinced that I was on the right lines, the diet on its own made very little difference.

I had made a friend at church called Moira who also had many health problems and we were convinced that she, too, had yeast infection. She decided to join me on the diet. One Sunday morning she came up to me and said, 'Guess what! My GP has become interested in yeast infection and he wants to meet you!'

This was incredible! I had thought it would be impossible ever to find a doctor who would be interested in what I had discovered, but now here was one wanting to discuss it with me. I made contact with him and we spent an interesting hour pooling our knowledge of candida. I arranged to transfer to his practice and he was very happy to prescribe an anti-fungal drug.

I began to feel extremely depressed and morbid. My sinuses and ears became painful. My arms, legs and back were aching all the time. I developed appalling pains in my gums which seemed to touch the nerve of every tooth, and searing pain which went right through the roof of my mouth. Some days the pain was so bad that I could not lift my face from the pillow. Things were getting worse rather than better.

I discovered that both garlic and yoghurt had anti-fungal properties, and I tried applying either or both of these to my mouth in an attempt to relieve the pain—with helpful but short-lived results. I painted my mouth with garlic oil each night before I went to bed. Praise God for a long-suffering husband!

This phase lasted several weeks, during which I continued to take the drug and kept strictly to the diet. Having come through the bad patch, things were just about the same as before. After a while, there seemed no point in continuing to take the anti-fungal drug so I just struggled on, still keeping to the diet, for another couple of years.

At Christmas 1987 I became ill with some sort of virus, and I just couldn't seem to get over it. Week after week, through the winter and early spring, I sat by the fire, aching all over and totally lacking energy. This was nothing new; it had been the pattern many times before. I would think all day about the breakfast dishes waiting to be cleared, but I just couldn't drag myself to do it. Occasionally I did, and then I would have to lean against the sink while the muscles all over my body were wracked with pain. For four months, it took more strength than I could muster to do that one small daily task.

In April I was still no better. I started thinking about others I knew, including Moira, who had problems very similar to mine. They were all much younger than me. Each one of us had been through many medical tests, but no answers had been found. I knew that the others had each come to believe that they had yeast infection too, and it occurred to me that, as Christians, we should be taking a stand together against our common enemy. After all, there is strength in numbers. Perhaps we could arrange to pray together once a week. They all agreed. The next Wednesday afternoon they came to my house and we prayed for each other and for an answer to our problems. We prayed that we might all be healed.

Within a week, we received the first part of the answer. Another friend lent me a back copy of a health magazine in which there was an appeal by some nutrition students for volunteers to take part in a research project. They were looking into the effectiveness of a natural substance called caprylic acid which was 'proving to be dramatically effective against the growing threat of *Candida albicans* infection'. The magazine was a few weeks old, but I quickly wrote off to see if I might still be in time to volunteer for the project.

Eventually I received a reply stating that sufficient volunteers had been found. That particular door was closed, but meanwhile I had done some detective work. I asked at every health food shop and pharmacy in my area if they had heard of a caprylic acid supplement. None had, for I later discovered that it was marketed by a very new company. However, it was eventually tracked down for me by a very kind pharmacist and I wrote off and asked for information.

I received in reply some interesting literature which explained that caprylic acid is a natural oil found in coconuts. It had been known for many years to have anti-fungal properties, and more recently its effect had been discovered as specific to *Candida albicans*. It had been available in Britain for only a few months. The information also included a recommendation to take supplements called probiotics which would help to restore friendly bacteria in the intestines.

I discovered that these two products together would cost quite a lot of money, even for an initial three weeks' supply. I discussed it with Robin, and we agreed that the timing was so extraordinary, following our prayer just a few days earlier, that it really did seem that God was showing the way he wanted us to go. We would therefore look to him for the financial resources as well.

I started taking the supplements. For three weeks nothing happened—and then it hit me. An enormous cloud of morbid depression descended, interspersed with bouts of severe anxiety. My ears became sore. I felt ill all over. I didn't know what was happening.

In the midst of all this, I had to face up to the fact that Robin was going away for three months. Some time previously, we had felt it right for him to apply to spend a term at Roffey Place Christian Training Centre in Sussex, at that time the base of Kingdom Faith Ministries. He was accepted, and arranged to have a term of unpaid leave from school. We calculated that we could just about afford it. We were both quite certain that this was what God wanted him to do, even though neither of us relished the idea of separation.

Being unwell all my life had made me very dependent, first on my parents and then on my husband, but I knew that God was telling me to learn to rely on him and to let Robin go to Roffey. Even so, I dreaded the thought of being alone, especially now that I was feeling so morbid and anxious.

The day arrived for Robin's departure. I woke up in the morning—and far from being full of dread, I felt an inexplicable sense of excitement! We had believed that God would bless our step of obedience, but I awoke that day *knowing* that something was already happening.

Within days of Robin going, several of my 'yeasty' friends asked if I could get hold of more of the supplements I was taking, for them to try themselves. Most of us had the same doctor, and he was very interested in what was going on.

We all started to get well. I managed to get to a church barn dance and one of my friends from the prayer group, whom I had only ever known as being 'limp' and pale, was dancing every dance. When I expressed surprise, she told me that she and her husband had cycled fifteen miles that day!

As my own health started to improve, people saw the change in me and began to ask if I could help them with their own health problems. I discovered a questionnaire which was a good way of telling whether or not someone had the symptoms of yeast infection. If they had a high score, I told them about the diet and the various supplements they needed. This all happened so quickly that, in Robin's second week away from home, I was staying up late every night in order to work out a book-keeping system for the money coming through my hands to pay for pots of anti-fungal capsules. I had very little time to miss my husband!

The real breakthrough came towards the end of June. Our younger daughter, Hannah, was at university in Cardiff and she was due home for the summer. Someone had to drive to Wales to collect her with all her belongings. Robin was away at Roffey so the someone had to be me. I had never in my life driven more than twenty miles without becoming fatigued. Now I was going to drive alone for over two hundred miles from Essex to Cardiff and back again.

In fact, with Hannah I drove to the Gower Peninsula and the Brecon Beacons and we spent a delightful couple of days walking together before driving back to Essex. On the way home we called in on Robin in Sussex. In four days I had driven over nine hundred miles; my health was fine, I wasn't even tired and I had enjoyed every minute. I even coped with a breakdown on the motorway! I felt better than I could ever remember feeling in my life before. While Robin was away at Roffey, we both learned important lessons and took major steps with God as we obeyed and trusted him—and we felt that a tap of blessing had been turned on in our lives.

When I first learned about *Candida albicans*, it was like finding a missing piece of a jigsaw puzzle. It explained so many things that had been going on in my body. I came to understand it like this: Living in the intestines of each one of us is a colony of microbes weighing about four pounds. It needs to have a correct balance of 'good guys' (ideally 80%) and 'bad guys' (20%) if we are to be healthy. Even the bad guys have a role to play, but they need to be kept under control in their 20% boundary, otherwise problems arise. One of these potential bad guys is the common yeast, *Candida albicans*.

Unfortunately, in this day and age we are doing almost everything possible to encourage our resident yeast to thrive. If you have ever made bread or wine, you will know that yeast is activated by sugar. Together they ferment and the yeast spreads. We now eat more sugar than any previous generation, much of it in tinned or packaged foods. In addition, refined grains like white flour quickly turn to glucose in the blood, adding to the sugar-load. This high amount of sugar 'feeds' the yeast in our intestines, encouraging it to thrive and spread.

At the same time, the over-use of antibiotics ensures that the good guys are depleted. Unfortunately these potential life-savers not only destroy the bug that made us ill, they also destroy the friendly bacteria so that the thriving yeast has more room to spread.

A third major factor which results in candida overgrowth is that any form of steroid treatment suppresses the immune system. It may have short-term, anti-inflammatory benefits, but in the long term you can be certain that immunity becomes weaker and weaker. People using steroid asthma puffers frequently have thrush in their mouth and throat for this very reason. Unfortunately, not many women realise that when they take the contraceptive pill or HRT, these too are steroid treatments. It is almost impossible to avoid a growing incidence of yeast infection after a few years on either the Pill or HRT—even though many women claim to feel wonderful at first. If only they knew that optimum nutrition provides better answers than hormone replacement therapy!

There are other reasons too, including a decline in breast-feeding, which is of course the best way to ensure that babies start life with a good level of friendly bacteria in their tummies. Without it, and particularly if the mother had vaginal thrush when giving birth, the baby is likely to develop candida problems, leading to colic, nappy rash, eczema, ear-ache—and possibly an asthma puffer by the age of five.

All these reasons, and others, mean that we are experiencing a situation which is fast becoming an epidemic, yet many doctors seem to be unaware of it. Fortunately some are aware, and a small but growing number of General Practitioners are happy for their candida patients to consult a good nutritionist.

When yeast gets out of control, it changes its shape from a spore to a fungal form. Under a microscope it looks very much like mould growing on an old piece of bread, with whiskery roots called mycelia sticking out of it. There is evidence that in this form it is able to penetrate the intestinal wall and invade the bloodstream. Once there, it can travel to any part of the body and set up a colony, causing problems which frequently are incorrectly diagnosed. For instance, a stubborn sore throat will probably be treated with several different antibiotics on the assumption that the infection is bacterial, but if this assumption is wrong and the infection is actually fungal, antibiotics will simply make the problem worse.

Candida causes problems in the digestive tract, like irritable bowel, constipation, diarrhoea, bloating and excessive wind. It can also invade any other tissue in the body: the urinary tract (causing kidney infections and cystitis); the sinuses, ears, mouth or throat (causing chronic pain and infection); the skin (causing acne, athlete's foot, eczema and psoriasis); the muscles (causing weakness, tremor, numbness, burning or tingling); the joints (causing multiple joint pain, stiffness and swelling); and vaginal tissue (causing irritation, soreness and discharge). One very common symptom is rectal irritation.

I discovered that candida seems to love to inhabit old injury sites such as knees or back; my repeated attacks of back pain from a spinal injury improved dramatically once the yeast was under control in my body.

In addition, candida in its fungal form releases poisons (seventy-nine have been identified!) which, among other things, cause mental or emotional symptoms—hence my bouts of depression and anxiety. Other common symptoms include a 'foggy' head, feelings of unreality, irritability, loss of memory, lack of concentration, drowsiness or insomnia.

Lack of energy, muscle weakness and fatigue can vary from being just slight and occasional right through to being constant and totally incapacitating.

Added to all this, the immune system uses so much strength in trying to hold back encroaching candida that it becomes too weak to deal with other invaders, so that allergies increase and infections take hold. Food allergy is very common in candida sufferers because, when candida burrows through the intestinal lining, it makes it leaky, so that little particles of incompletely-digested protein from our food are able to enter the bloodstream, causing the immune system to react.

Inhaled allergens also become a problem. Things like paint and household cleaners create a nightmare of symptoms, physical and mental. Domestic gas and petrol fumes can do the same. Some people react dreadfully to perfumes and after-shave, playing havoc with their love-life! And I discovered that there were actually other people like me who had become allergic to anaesthetics, in spite of the fact that one hospital consultant told me that this was just not possible and that I was obviously the type of woman who fainted when she saw the needle! (I couldn't help wondering how he would cope if he had to have three teeth crowned in one go without an anaesthetic, as I once did!)

In women, candida interferes with hormone function causing menstrual problems, premenstrual syndrome and even infertility. They may have violent mood swings. Men are just as susceptible as women but it most frequently affects their digestive systems giving rise to bloating, wind or irritable bowel, and frequently it leads to depression or a foul temper! Candida is contagious and so can be transferred through sexual contact.

A 'yeasty' person may suffer from either just a few or else a whole host of different symptoms. The difference between candidiasis and an illness like flu or a throat infection is that it's persistent—either continuous or recurring at frequent intervals. Apart from thrush in the mouth or vagina, there is often nothing to be seen so the condition is difficult to diagnose and many sufferers have to bear the loneliness of being misunderstood and the indignity of being regarded as a hypochondriac. Being told that your symptoms are 'all in your mind' is of no help to anyone.

Even so, when I first discovered that there was one basic underlying cause of all my health problems, it was a great relief. For years I had felt that I was disintegrating in all directions—falling apart at the seams! Now I knew that there was just one condition for which I needed the answer—and which, in time, God gave. Eventually I realised that I had been led to put together a successful four-point plan (for fuller detail, see Appendix D):

1. Anti-candida diet (see Appendix E).
2. A tailor-made programme of vitamins and minerals to boost immunity.
3. Natural anti-fungals, like caprylic acid from coconuts.

4. Supplements providing friendly bacteria (acidophilus
   and bifidobacteria).

All four points are essential in the candida battle; omitting
just one will lead to failure.

When I later trained at the Institute for Optimum
Nutrition, I learned the underlying biochemical reasons for
the effectiveness of the four-point plan, and this increased my
confidence in passing it on to other people. As I did so, I saw
many regain their health. It takes time, patience, determination—and faith. For most people it takes many months to get
well, but each person is so different and there are so many
factors involved that my initial reply to the question, 'How
long will it take?' can only be 'How long is a piece of string?'

Yeast infection is a wretched business from beginning to
end, for even the process of getting rid of it is no joy-ride.
Dead yeast releases even more poisons than when it is alive,
and these have to be dealt with and off-loaded by the liver.
Meanwhile, as they circulate round the body, they play
havoc. They can cause a flare-up of all your old symptoms,
so that for a while you might feel you are getting worse rather
than better, just as I did. They can make you ache all over
and, perhaps worst of all, they can make you feel really
anxious or depressed. This is known as 'die-off' reaction (or
Herxheimer's reaction) and during these times you have to
hold on in faith and praise the Lord, because it means that
yeast is being destroyed so that in fact you are getting better,
even though you might feel dreadful!

There is quite a lot that can be done to regulate and
control the severity of this die-off reaction but, even so, you
need to know in advance that the going might be tough at
times. But, praise God, it doesn't last like this for ever and
you *do* get well. I did!

If you suspect that you might have candida, I suggest that

you complete the candida score sheet in Appendix C and then try the anti-candida diet (Appendix E). If you feel worse, you are on the right track. This is your first experience of die-off reaction. Take heart because, after the initial month, many people feel better than they have in years.

But, be warned! Anyone entering this battlefield will possibly find themselves in a minefield of confusion and depression caused by die-off toxins, so praying friends are needed and also someone, possibly a nutritionist, who can give objective advice and be supportive and encouraging.

Remember, Father God knows exactly what you have been through and what you are enduring right now. He will not let you go, but he is asking you to play a responsible part in destroying the fungal invaders in your body by embarking on a diet which involves firm self-discipline, perseverance and determination.

Go on, you can do it! Join with Paul in saying, 'I can do everything through him who gives me strength' (Philippians 4:13).

Wise Words

'You must destroy all the peoples the Lord your God gives over to you. Do not look on them with pity and do not serve their gods for that will be a snare to you'
(Deuteronomy 7:16).

For Action

- **Complete the candida score sheet** (Appendix C) and when you know your total score be guided by the relevant comment.
- **Study the four-point plan** (Appendix D) and the anti-candida diet (Appendix E).

- **Pray for motivation and will-power** to make changes to your diet and follow it *totally*. Get your friends praying, too.
- **Start to restock your kitchen** with appropriate, healthy foods and look for suitable recipes (see Appendix F). Decide on a day to start the diet, then *do it*.
- **Work out an appropriate vitamin/mineral programme** See *The Optimum Nutrition Bible* by Patrick Holford (Piatkus) or consult a nutritionist for a tailor-made programme. Take your vitamins regularly.
- A month after starting the diet and vitamins, if you feel on a reasonably even keel, **introduce caprylic acid supplements.** Start with a low level and build up gradually, allowing at least five days at each level.
- **At the same time, start taking two acidophilus supplements** every day.
- **Give away your house-plants**—you are breathing in airborne mould spores from the soil!
- **Drink lots of water and increase Vitamin C** if necessary to off-load die-off toxins. Take enough each day to encourage a loose bowel motion. Never increase caprylic acid if you are experiencing unpleasant die-off symptoms.
- **If problems persist, or progress seems stuck, you really need a nutritionist's advice.** You might have food allergies confusing the picture, or your liver might need some help to cope with toxins. These and other situations can all be helped.
- **Recognise each bout of die-off as a step closer to healing.**
- **Pray some more!**

CHAPTER 11

WHY ME?—CHRONIC FATIGUE SYNDROME

'In all their affliction he was afflicted, and he personally saved them. In his love and pity he redeemed them and lifted them up and carried them through all the years'
(Isaiah 63:9, *Living Bible*).

Not long after I had qualified as a nutrition consultant, I was contacted by Christine, wife of a Scottish Army chaplain. Since having glandular fever at the age of twenty, Christine's health had never been stable, although previously she had been very fit and active with a love of sailing. Life as an army wife meant constant moves and, after having four babies, she described herself as an 'exhausted heap', being weakened even further by frequent viral infections.

In 1990, her husband was away serving in the Gulf War and Christine's exhaustion became unbearable. At first she thought it was the stress of coping alone with four young children and the worry of having her husband in a war zone, but then she developed intense pains in her back and neck, together with deterioration in vision and concentration. An army doctor diagnosed ME (Myalgic encephalomyelitis) which Christine did not accept until she became almost totally bed-ridden and could hardly brush her hair. Another doctor confirmed the diagnosis and one day Christine contacted me for help. She was thirty-nine years old.

I had already come to realise that ME is basically a problem of an overloaded and broken-down immune system, caused by a variable combination of factors. In Christine's case, these appeared to be viral infection, hypoglycaemia (low blood sugar), food intolerance, stress, lifestyle factors, toxicity from amalgam fillings, nutritional deficiencies and yeast infection (candidiasis).

Christine had been taking a contraceptive pill, a sure way of encouraging candida activity because of its steroid activity which suppresses immunity. I explained to her (by post and telephone) my nutritional approach for strengthening immunity which took into account recommendations for regulating blood sugar, overcoming allergies, destroying candida, etc., and she started on the recommended diet and supplements. Almost immediately she had a blinding headache as she broke her addiction to tea, coffee and chocolate, but after three days she found she was stronger than before. Christmas came and Christine relaxed the diet. As a result, she spent ten days feeling worse than she had for a year. She needed no further persuasion of the benefits of a candida-starving diet!

Her hopes were set on taking the whole family to America for a Christian conference in six months' time—and she made it! She had all the energy she needed for six weeks of seminars and travel. She looked and felt so well that no one guessed she had a health problem. Staying with various families made it impossible to keep to the diet but there were no ill-effects until just towards the end when she noticed a few returning symptoms, so on the whole she was very encouraged.

Once home she returned to the programme and experienced phases of alternating migraine and increased well-being as candida which had been slightly reactivated was once more brought under control. Her next nutritional analysis showed excellent improvements in blood sugar control, premenstrual symptoms, resting pulse rate and weight loss. Her candida score had fallen considerably, but she was determined to make sure that it was fully under control.

Christine become so convinced of the value of nutritional therapy that she is now a nutritionist herself!

My files are full of similar case histories. Let me tell you about Fiona.

Fiona, aged nineteen and a lovely Christian girl, had been diagnosed with chronic Post Viral Fatigue Syndrome (another name sometimes given to ME) seven months before she contacted me. She was consulting a neurologist who had prescribed antidepressants. She had been too ill to continue her first year at university but, having consulted me in January, she was fully fit and able to resume her studies in the autumn term. This is her own account, written the following Christmas:

Having collapsed in a university lecture, I was told I would be ill for about two weeks. I waited with great frustration, only to find that three months later I still could not even walk. I had no memory or concentration. Despite feeling exhausted, I could never sleep until the early hours of the morning, and then would wake feeling as though I had run a marathon! I could not cope with light, noise or conversation. I had so many blood tests, the nurses joked that I might 'dry up'!

In pain and bed-ridden, I wondered what was happening to my body. Glandular fever was then diagnosed but a few months later I was feeling even weaker. I struggled to get back to university but only managed two lectures in a whole term. I couldn't manage stairs and when I first went to the supermarket I just wanted to lie down in the middle of the aisle. My muscles still ached, especially when I used them!

Finally, I saw a neurologist who gave me a brain scan and told me I had a classic case of ME. He confirmed that my brain did actually exist but that it was working like a 'faulty computer programme'! The university tried to encourage me to take a year out to recover. I eventually gave in and later discovered Erica's nutritional regime and the anti-candida diet. My headaches immediately disappeared. I had forgotten what life was like without them. From then on, my symptoms gradually left.

I am now relaxing the diet, having been on it for a year, and have completed a term back at university (including a game of hockey and an all-night ball!). Friends are amazed at the speed of my recovery and it feels so good to have my health back. I have been challenged by the amount of sugar I was consuming. The diet has been the key to my recovery, along with the prayers of many friends. I have been really blessed and my eyes have been opened to the basic fact that what we eat will hugely affect our health and general well-being.

This story has a particularly happy ending, because Fiona gained a first in her degree.

In Britain alone, over 150,000 people are reckoned to be suffering from Chronic Fatigue Syndrome, or ME. These are the diagnosed cases; countless others are struggling with an illness which has not even been given a name. Typical ME symptoms include unrelenting fatigue, lethargy, aches and pains, 'woolly' head, poor memory, digestive problems (including irritable bowel and bloating), shivering or sweating, mood swings, anxiety, depression, irritability, PMT and loss of weight control, to name just a few! To receive a formal medical diagnosis of ME or CFS, symptoms must have been present for six months or longer.

Yet I stick my neck out and say that I believe there is no such thing as ME. What I mean by this is that symptoms vary from person to person (apart from fatigue, the common denominator), and there are many different causes—so there is not just one condition which can be given just one label. Detective work is needed to identify specific situations which are responsible for the symptoms.

Back in my mid-thirties, for a whole year my health was even worse than usual. I was weak, sick and aching, unable to care for my family. Today, almost certainly I would have been diagnosed with ME—but we discovered eventually that I was reacting to the new North Sea gas. That particular load on my immune system was allergy, and gas had to go from the house. Struggling with unsuspected candida and low blood sugar, my immune system was so severely overloaded that it had eventually broken down and my life had become a struggle to get through each day and night.

So ME is made up of an overwhelming array of symptoms and causes. Does Scripture say anything to bring hope? I believe it does.

> You may say to yourselves, 'These nations are stronger than we are: how can we drive them out?' But do not be afraid of them; remember well what the Lord your God did to Pharaoh and to all Egypt . . . The Lord your God will do the same to all the peoples you now fear
>
> (Deuteronomy 7:17–19).

And I knew without any doubt that this was God's promise to me.

In my book *ME: Sailing Free*, I describe the immune system as a ship which is carrying a whole load of cargo. It sails along well until it hits a rock which makes a hole in its side, and then the weight of the cargo pushes the hole below the water-line, water pours in and the ship begins to sink. However, if the heaviest pieces of cargo can be identified and removed before the ship has sunk too far, this will lighten the load on board so that the hole stays above the water-line and the ship stays afloat. Below are listed ten common pieces of cargo, any of which will weigh down the good ship 'Immunity'!:

1. Viral infection, past or present.
2. Allergy—food or environmental.
3. Nutritional deficiencies.
4. Toxicity, poor liver function.
5. Lifestyle.
6. Stress, exhausted adrenal glands.
7. Hyperventilation.
8. Underactive thyroid.
9. Low blood sugar.
10. Unbalanced intestinal microbes—candida overgrowth, parasites.

Much emphasis is placed by medical researchers on trying to find a virus, but hundreds of success stories have convinced me that this is the wrong direction to take. What is important is to discover the factors which have led to the weakened immunity which has allowed a possible virus to take hold—and then do something about them.

For instance, Epstein-Barr is the name of a virus which is commonly found in ME sufferers. However, it is equally commonly found in people who are not ill. The deciding factor as to whether or not someone succumbs to such a virus is their own susceptibility—in other words, whether or not their immune system has strength to fight it off. A strong ship which has very few or even no pieces of cargo on board will stay afloat even if it crashes onto a rock and gets a hole in the side. There is no weight on board to push the hole below the water-line.

Quite a few possible pieces of cargo are discussed in other parts of this book. For those which are not, nutritional therapy still plays an invaluable part. Once all the pieces of cargo have been removed so that health can be restored, it makes sense to take responsibility for our future health by ensuring that our immune systems and all other parts of the body continue to work as efficiently as possible. And how can we do this? Through optimum nutrition!

A final word—it is never too late and you are never too old! My book *ME: Sailing Free* contains the testimony of a lady aged ninety-one. She had suffered for several years from chronic fatigue (ME), sinusitis, thrush and gout. A year after starting on an appropriate nutritional regime, she was able to write the following:

After a year's faithful adherence to all your suggestions and recommendations, I feel a completely different person. The gout in my feet has completely gone; the catarrah in my ear, which had prevented me from hearing, is definitely clearing up and I no longer wear a hearing aid. I am beginning to catch up with all the jobs I should have done long ago in my capacity as manager of a block of thirty-two flats. I also do all my own shopping and cooking and all the other things necessary to keep alive.

Not a bad recovery at the age of ninety-one!

God's plan for our lives is that we should continue to be fruitful, right into a ripe old age. Even if along the way we have lost some years to sickness, let's determine to co-operate with God, and look forward to being active in our nineties!

Wise Words

*'They will still bear fruit in old age, they will stay fresh
and green, proclaiming, "The Lord is upright; he is my
Rock, and there is no wickedness in him"'*
(Psalm 92:14).

For Action

- **Carefully read the chapters in this book which refer
  to possible pieces of cargo** weighing down your immune
  system: Chapter 8 (low blood sugar), Chapter 9 (allergy),
  Chapter 10 (candida), Chapter 17 (toxicity), Chapter 18
  (stress).

- As you read, **ask God for words of knowledge** to guide
  you to root causes of your illness, and then ask for words of
  wisdom so that you know what to do about them.

- **Ask him also for the gift of faith** that you will be well. At
  the same time, accept the situation as it is at this moment, so
  that you are in a place of peace and trust and not in anger or
  frustration. **Read faith-building books like *God's Plan
  for Your Healing* by Colin Urquhart (Hodder &
  Stoughton).**

- **Read the Bible for all you're worth** and ask God to guide
  you to specific verses which will build your faith.

- **Trust and pray—but also be obedient,** and be prepared
  to make changes to your eating habits if this is what God asks
  of you! (See Appendix E.)

CHAPTER 12

UNPEACEFUL HEARTS— CARDIOVASCULAR DISEASE

'A heart at peace gives life to the body' (Proverbs 14:30).

One evening, fairly late, the doorbell rang and David stood on our step. He had recently joined our church and we had got to know him a little. He apologised for calling unexpectedly and explained that as he was driving home, it had entered his mind to call on us. He decided that if there was a parking space reasonably close to our house, he would pull in and just see if we happened to be free. There was a space right by our gate!

We were surprised but pleased to see him, and we sat and chatted over a hot drink. David showed an interest in the nutrition work we were doing and after a while he asked if nutrition might be helpful for a heart condition.

'Almost certainly,' I said, 'because when you give the body the nutrients it needs to correct any biochemical imbalances or deficiencies, it will often do amazing things to sort itself out. Having said this, it is impossible to guarantee how much might be achieved. Why do you ask?'

We then learned that David had undergone major by-pass surgery eleven years before. His health since then had been passable but he had to attend hospital for frequent check-ups. He thought perhaps it might be a good idea to ask me to prepare a nutritional programme for him, and he said he would give it some thought and probably get back to us about it in due course. Then he went home.

The next morning at nine o'clock we received a telephone call from the headmaster of the school where David taught. He said that David had been rushed to hospital in the middle of the night with heart pains and that he had asked for us to be told and had made a request that, if possible, we might visit him.

When our work for the day was over, Robin and I set off for the hospital—and were greatly relieved to find that David was not too seriously ill; the pains in the night had thankfully been no more than a warning. However, David was taking it very seriously, and he was quite convinced that God had prompted him to visit us the previous evening—and had even made a parking space available—so that he could find out how to improve the health of his heart. He had vaguely considered having a nutritional consultation at some time in the future, but this had now assumed a greater degree of urgency. He said, 'I want to do whatever you tell me!' And he did.

Three months later, a heart specialist at the hospital was so amazed at the improvements in David's health that he thought he had picked up the wrong file! David did eventually die, but not before he had led ten more very active years, well into his retirement, during which he conducted choirs and orchestras on international tours, helped at Christian camps for schools and even led school ski trips. He faithfully took what he liked to call his 'pink pills for pale people'—the vitamins and minerals which, together with changes in diet, helped to give his heart a whole new lease of life.

Proverbs 14:30 says, 'A heart at peace gives life to the

body.' Of course, I realise that this is referring to peace of mind, but it is equally true that the physical heart gives life to the body because it is the pump for the bloodstream which carries oxygen and vital nutrients to all our cells. If the heart has *dis*-ease, there *is* no life in the body!

Statistically, the heart is in pretty poor shape. No less than half of us can expect to develop heart disease; heart attacks are experienced by one in four men before retirement age and of these one in four will actually die before the age of sixty-five. Heart disease has reached epidemic proportions far higher than those of AIDS, yet in the 1930s it was so rare that doctors found it difficult to diagnose. That's the bad news. The good news is that in the vast majority of cases it is totally preventable and avoidable. Want to know more?

Heart disease should really be called disease of the arteries. Arteries are blood vessels, or transport channels, which carry everything that is needed to every cell in the body—oxygen, fuel, building materials, vitamins and minerals. The blood circulation is central to life. Tiny blood vessels absorb oxygen from the lungs and carry it to arteries which take it to the heart, which in turn pumps it to the cells. Waste products from the cells are carried back to the lungs to be breathed out as carbon dioxide, and to the kidneys to be off-loaded in urine.

Arteries can suffer from a build-up of 'gunge' or plaque (the medical term is atheroma, which is the Greek word for porridge!). It is not hard to visualise that such a build-up will narrow the channel through which blood is flowing. If, at the same time, the blood becomes too thick, a clot may develop which causes a block in the narrowed artery. The heart is deprived of oxygen, resulting in a heart attack. Angina indicates a partial block.

If a block occurs in arteries entering the head, oxygen

cannot reach the brain and the result is a stroke; if a block occurs in the legs, it causes thrombosis. The situation appears to develop as damage is caused to the artery walls. This may be due to dangerous molecules known as free radicals, many of which are produced by eating fried or burnt foods or by smoking, or it may be due to a substance called homocysteine. Local cells then proliferate in an attempt to repair the damage, forming plaque by attracting cholesterol, fats and calcium from the blood. Thus the channel is narrowed down and may easily be blocked by blood which is too thick and forms into clots, or by pieces of plaque breaking off the artery wall.

Cholesterol is not quite the bad guy we've been led to believe! Among other things, it is needed for the efficient working of our brains, nerves and hormones. But it needs to be carried to its various sites and it is the balance of the carriers which is important. The bad carriers, known as LDLs (Low Density Lipoproteins) tend to dump cholesterol inside the arteries, whereas the good carriers, known as HDLs (High Density Lipoproteins) help to remove it. Cholesterol only appears to play a part in increasing the risk of heart disease once damage has already occurred to the artery walls, and it then becomes attracted to that place—presumably in a misguided attempt to patch it up!

The theory that homocysteine causes initial damage to the artery walls has recently been well confirmed by research. Homocysteine is a toxic substance produced by a certain type of protein in the diet. It is mostly found in meat. However, if we receive good levels of Vitamins B6, B12 and folic acid from our diet, it is converted into a totally harmless substance. Unfortunately, the diets of a great many people provide only very low levels of these necessary vitamins, if any! High levels of homocysteine in the blood have been found to cause a greatly increased risk of heart disease, and a really high level (as found in 20% of 1,500 people who were monitored) is shown to double the risk.

Those most at risk are high meat-eaters with a low intake of green leafy vegetables, nuts, whole grains, wheatgerm, fish and free-range chicken, all good sources of Vitamin B6 and folic acid. A hamburger diet is therefore a high risk for heart disease because it is high in protein, high in saturated fat, high in cholesterol and almost completely lacking in B6 and folic acid.

Apart from deposits in the arteries and thickening (or clotting) of the blood, there is a third factor involved in so-called heart disease, which is hardening of the artery walls, when they lose their elasticity. Imagine a rubber hose-pipe with the water-tap turned full on, causing maximum pressure—that is your bloodstream with your heart pumping its hardest, and it is measured by the top figure (systolic) of your blood pressure. The bottom figure (diastolic) is when the tap is turned off and the pressure is at its lowest, as the heart takes a rest between beats. If the hose-pipe is furred up or the water is full of bits, or if the pipe is made of steel instead of rubber, the pressure will be higher—just as it will if your arteries are full of plaque or if your blood is thick and clotted or if your artery walls have hardened.

High blood pressure is a significant risk-factor for heart disease, showing that something is wrong with the arteries, but unfortunately it gives no symptoms to warn us that trouble is looming.

It is generally accepted that blood pressure rises with age, but there is no reason why this should be the case. Increased blood pressure is an indication that more things are going wrong with the cardiovascular system but this is not necessarily age-related. Unfortunately, doctors generally take the average patient to be the norm because they so seldom have the pleasure of seeing someone who is optimally nourished and whose body is working really efficiently!

When I was training to be a nutritionist and learning about blood pressure, at fifty-three years old my own reading was 140/90. I knew my doctor would think this was fine because the systolic reading is accepted as being 100 plus your age; in other words, mine would have been acceptable if it had been 153, whereas in fact it was 140. The diastolic figure of 90 was just about borderline but the systolic was absolutely fine. This was encouraging, but I decided to practise what I was learning to preach and see if I could reduce it. After three months of taking appropriate nutritional supplements, my blood pressure reading had fallen to 108/68, and it is usually not far from those figures some eleven years later on.

So what are the most important things you should do to reduce your blood pressure and avoid the risk of heart disease? Thin the blood, reduce free radical activity and damage, disarm the dangerous homocysteine, encourage good carriers for cholesterol, increase elasticity to artery walls and clean out the rubbish inside them. And all this can be achieved through good nutrition! It is true to say that the horrors of heart disease are largely preventable and frequently reversible simply by making some changes to your diet and your lifestyle and taking a few food supplements. This has to be good news!

Here are some interesting facts about the role of various nutrients in preventing disease of the heart and arteries:

- Vitamins A, C, E and selenium are antioxidants which combat free radicals.
- Antioxidants and the amino acid lysine, also the essential

fatty acids in fish oil and in flax seed (linseed), help to keep blood thin, stop a build-up of plaque in the arteries and even reverse the process.

- Vitamin C can stop hardening of the arteries, reduce clotting, remove cholesterol and increase elasticity of artery walls.

- Vitamin E helps to transport cholesterol, prevents clotting, helps dissolve existing clots, reduces blood stickiness and helps cells to use oxygen (important in angina).

- Vitamin B3 (niacin) and fish oils help to remove cholesterol by encouraging healthy HDL carriers.

- Vitamins B6, B12 and folic acid prevent homocysteine from damaging artery walls.

- Zinc, calcium and Vitamin C help to off-load lead and cadmium, toxic metals which cause an increase in blood pressure.

- Calcium, potassium, magnesium, Vitamin B3 and Vitamin B6 (a natural diuretic) help to reduce blood pressure.

- Co-enzyme Q10 and the amino acid Taurine can help to reduce high blood pressure which has resisted other methods.

- Magnesium is needed to avoid cramping of the arteries which feed the heart muscle (a deficiency can cause a heart attack even without a blockage in the artery).

Wise Words

'A happy heart makes the face cheerful' (Proverbs 15:13).

For Action

- **Avoid six Ss**—salt, sugar, saturated fat, stimulants, stress and smoking.

- **You don't need added salt,** but if you miss it you are probably zinc-deficient.
- **You don't need sugar.** Show your sweet tooth who is boss!
- **You don't need saturated (mainly animal) fat but you do need fish oils and seed oils,** so eat plenty of salmon, herring, mackerel, tuna and sardines (Eskimos don't have heart disease!) and good quality seed oils (sunflower, sesame, flax), or eat the seeds themselves, whole or ground.
- **Stimulants to avoid are sugar, chocolate, cola, tea and coffee.** (Try Rooibosch, Barleycup or herb teas.)
- **Stress increases blood pressure** by constricting blood vessels and causing the heart to beat faster. Note what makes you tense; bring it to God and learn to leave it with him.
- **Stop smoking.** It starves cells of oxygen and thickens blood. Twice as many smokers die of heart disease than of lung cancer.
- **Take a good supplement programme;** if you are concerned to get it right, see a nutritionist.
- **Lose some weight if you need to.**
- **Take exercise**—brisk walking, cycling, swimming, aerobics—at least three times a week for at least twenty minutes.
- **Choose to eat wisely** for the health of your heart. (See Appendix G.)

CHAPTER 13

TURBULENT TUMMIES—DIGESTIVE DISORDERS

'The churning inside me never stops, days of suffering confront me' (Job 30:27).

When Catherine came to see me, she told me she had been unable to teach for the past term because of the terrible state of her tummy. She had diarrhoea all the time, needing to run to the lavatory as many as thirteen times every day, and she frequently passed quite large amounts of blood. The condition had been diagnosed as ulcerative colitis and she was due to have an operation in three weeks' time to remove part of her colon. She wondered if I could suggest anything to help.

Faced with such a severe situation, I confess that my mind was daunted by the challenge but I was certainly happy to see if anything might possibly bring her some short-term relief. I formulated a nutritional programme for her, recommending changes in her diet and supplements to take. She followed my advice to the letter; she was prepared to do absolutely anything. The supplements contained a variety of nutrients needed to heal and strengthen the intestinal wall, while at the same time improving her overall nutritional status.

I think that I was probably more amazed than Catherine when, quite quickly, both the diarrhoea and the bleeding stopped and, although she went into hospital as arranged, the surgeon decided that an operation was no longer necessary. Catherine was a Christian so together we gave glory to God.

Another Christian, Jane, contacted me with severe indigestion and an appallingly acidic and painful stomach. An ulcer had been suspected but medical investigations had found nothing. Jane herself was convinced that she must have a parasite, possibly Helicobacter pylori, but once again test reports were negative. Antacid medications prescribed by her doctor simply made the situation a great deal worse, increasing the pain to such an extent that she was unable to sleep.

I had little doubt that at least part of Jane's problem was due to an overgrowth of yeast in her intestines (as described in Chapter 10), but I was puzzled by the tremendous amount of burning acidity which caused her to be in so much agony. She frequently rang in the mornings, after a particularly bad night, with a desperate plea for help.

I then discovered that Jane had been trying to control her blood pressure and cholesterol levels by drinking cider vinegar and honey. These conditions were also being treated by a doctor but she had experienced bad side-effects to the initial medication he prescribed so another drug was tried. The doctor told her to stop taking cider vinegar because it would be counter-productive. However, cholesterol levels rose and, in a panic, Jane returned to her cider vinegar and honey. She took it for well over a year.

She received prayer ministry at her church, and after that every blood pressure reading was normal, indicating that she had received a very definite healing from God, so she stopped the medication but still continued to take the cider vinegar.

She was worried by the fact that she frequently coughed up what she described as 'white froth', but otherwise she was reasonably well until just a few weeks before she contacted me. One night, she had eaten a Chinese meal and that is when the acidity and pain had started. Since then she had been unable to lie down in bed at night because of the tremendous amount of burning acid which rose up in her gullet, causing severe pain.

I was even more firmly convinced that Jane had an overgrowth of yeast. Drinking neat vinegar every day for a year would certainly have encouraged it, as would any other fermented product. In addition, the honey she mixed with the vinegar would also have encouraged candida to thrive because yeast 'feeds' on any type of sugar, including natural fructose. While trying to find a natural way of curing her high blood pressure, Jane had been giving her resident yeast a bean-feast!

The last straw would have come when she ate a Chinese meal because almost certainly it was flavoured with monosodium glutamate, which is a product of yeast, as well as with soy sauce, which is fermented. 'Yeasty' people often fall into a trap with this type of food and suffer the consequences without knowing why. To me, it was fairly obvious that, since the Chinese meal, the yeast in Jane's stomach and intestines had completely taken over. Among other things, it was causing fermentation whenever she ate anything which was even slightly sweet, forming the white froth which she noticed when she coughed.

The first thing I advised Jane to do was to mix some Slippery Elm powder with water and drink it before each meal, because this would provide a protective covering for

the inflamed walls of her digestive tract which had been traumatised by so much acid vinegar and fermentation. I also
advised her to take digestive enzymes to support all her
digestive processes, and I put her on the anti-candida diet.
After three weeks she reported having no indigestion and the
foaming mucus had lessened, but she still experienced acidic
burning.

About six weeks into the programme, Jane reported that
she was very much better. The Slippery Elm had settled her
stomach well, she had been able to take the vitamins and
minerals which I had recommended and she was about to
start taking anti-fungal supplements to destroy candida as
well as supplements to reintroduce friendly bacteria into her
digestive tract, as I had advised.

Jane persevered with her regime and after another three
months she was able to report that the acid stomach and
indigestion had completely gone away. Many other minor
symptoms had also cleared, including insomnia, irritability,
poor concentration and sore throat. Jane realised that she
had largely brought her problems upon herself by trying to
treat the high blood pressure without having proper nutritional advice, and by ignoring the doctor's instruction to
stop taking the cider vinegar and honey. She felt she had to
repent to God for her stubbornness, and perhaps this paved
the way for his healing in her body.

The situations I have described are just two of many ways
in which things can go wrong in the digestive tract. For the
most part, it puts up with an awful lot of abuse but there
comes a 'last straw' situation when it just has to cry out for
help.

When we think of our tummies, we tend to think of them
as being 'inside' us. In fact, the digestive tract is a long tube
which is a continuation of our external skin. Our real

'insides' are made up of cells, muscles, fibres, organs, nerves, glands, flesh, bones and blood which are packed neatly between the two layers of our outside skin and the walls of the digestive tract. The digestive tube itself is open to the world at both ends! It measures about thirty feet in length and its surface area, if spread out, would measure roughly the size of a tennis court.

The purpose of the digestive tract is to convert the food we eat into tiny particles which can be absorbed through its wall to nourish our cells. At the same time, the wall cleverly acts as a barrier to prevent toxins and bacteria from entering our bloodstream. It very skilfully distinguishes between what should and should not be allowed to pass through. Amazingly, the lining of a healthy digestive tract replaces itself every few days.

Efficient digestion is essential for nutrients to be absorbed and taken into the cells of our bodies. It is also important for the efficient elimination of toxins. Things can go wrong at any point along the way, on the long journey from the mouth to the rectum via the oesophagus, stomach and small and large intestines. Other organs which are directly involved with digestion are the salivary glands, liver, gall-bladder and pancreas.

Various situations can make the intestinal wall become leaky, which means that it is no longer a barrier against toxins, bacteria or incompletely-digested food. These microbes and particles are then able to enter the bloodstream and gain entry into our cells, causing various problems. For instance, the immune system will react to undigested food particles so a leaky gut is a major cause of food sensitivities.

It is all too common, unfortunately, to suffer from problems of the digestive tract. Mouth ulcers, indigestion, flatulence, heartburn, nausea, stomach pains, gastritis, ulcers, gall-bladder disease, irritable bowel syndrome, bloating, diarrhoea, constipation, colitis, diverticulitis, spastic colon—the list goes on!

One of the main causes of digestive problems is an imbalance of bacteria which live in the tube—of which there are about a hundred trillion, weighing together about four pounds. There are actually more bacteria in our intestinal tract than there are cells in our entire body, and there are up to five hundred different types of them.

The importance of the correct balance of these bacteria you have already seen in Chapter 10, where an overgrowth of candida was described as being one of the potential 'bad guys' let loose. There are other bad guys too, and as these all proliferate and grow stronger, the good guys are pushed back, becoming weaker and allowing even more bad guys to take hold.

There was a time when parasite infections were associated mainly with contamination of food or water in countries where the climate is hot and the hygiene poor. Nowadays it is increasingly common for an efficient laboratory test to be able to find at least one type of parasite in a stool specimen. A parasite might be harboured for years without causing symptoms, but if a second bad guy comes on the scene, such as *Candida albicans*, it triggers the parasite into action and the adverse effects of them both become pronounced. Add to the picture a 'leaky gut' and the parasite can freely enter the bloodstream, leading to severe ill health for which the cause is frequently not suspected.

There are some very detailed laboratory tests available based on stool and urine analysis which can be extremely helpful. Such tests are quite expensive but people who have them invariably feel that they are worth every penny if the root cause of their illness is at last discovered, because then it can be tackled in appropriate ways.

An imbalance of microbes in the digestive tract is known as 'gut dysbiosis'. It has many causes including stress, antibiotics, steroids, painkillers, X-rays, low levels of stomach acid, constipation and, of course, poor diet. Our Western diet, high in sugar, fat and processed foods, not only encourages the bad-guy microbes to thrive but fails to provide enough nutrients to allow the body to repair itself and stay in working order.

One of the most common diet-related problems in the digestive tract is indigestion—which many people seem to think is due to a deficiency of indigestion tablets because they take them all the time! Since indigestion is frequently caused by a deficiency of stomach acid, rather than too much, antacid preparations simply make matters worse. They also increase body levels of aluminium which is a toxic mineral but the major ingredient of many indigestion 'remedies'.

Diverticulitis is a bowel disease which causes many people to suffer immense pain and the eventual loss of part of their bowel, frequently necessitating a colostomy. Yet diverticulitis is virtually unknown in countries where they do not eat our Western diet, because its cause is the chronic constipation which is encouraged by low-fibre foods. You could say that diverticulitis is caused by a lifetime of eating white flour—in bread, pastry, cakes, pasta and biscuits—because this type of low-fibre food creates the wrong consistency for the efficient movement of material needing to be moved through the digestive tract by automatic muscular contractions known as peristalsis. A build-up of waste products then takes place, which encourages little pockets to be pushed out in the wall of the bowel and these become a collection point for the putrefying remains of food and for bacteria. Sometimes one of the little pockets will burst, releasing life-threatening toxins into the bloodstream, so immediate surgery is vital. Yet all this would never happen if we ate brown flour instead of white and made a few other basic changes to our diets.

There are various nutritional and herbal supplements which can help to heal a leaky, inflamed or ulcerated intestinal wall or destroy unfriendly bacteria or parasites and build up the 'good guys' in the gut. But none of these interventions will bring lasting benefit without a determined attempt to make radical changes in eating habits.

Faulty digestion and absorption and any type of abnormal gut reactions create chaos in every system and process of the body, interfering with immunity, the brain and nervous system, the heart and circulatory system, energy production, glandular and hormonal function and liver function, the last of these affecting the body's ability to eliminate toxins. Getting it right leads to good levels of energy and stamina, a stronger heart and immune system, an alert mind, happy hormones and a clear, healthy skin—in fact, all the benefits of nutrition as God intended!

Wise Words

'Worship the Lord your God, and his blessing will be on your food and water' (Exodus 23:25).

For Action

• **Make sure you are relaxed when you eat, and chew your food well.** Digestion of carbohydrates (vegetables, grains, fruit) starts in the mouth and is continued in the small intestine, while digestion of protein starts in the stomach.

Undigested food putrefies and causes flatulence, bloating, indigestion, bad breath, food allergies and lack of energy.

- **Read Appendix M—Guidelines for Healthy Eating.** Don't be confused by apparently acid foods—it's what they become once digested that matters.
- **Read Appendix H for advice on diverticulitis and other problems of the bowel.**
- **Don't take antacid pills or medicines.** They will make the situation worse! Try taking digestive enzyme supplements at the start of every meal. If this doesn't bring sufficient relief, do a beetroot test to show whether your stomach is producing too little or too much acid (the symptoms of each are exactly the same!) Eat some beetroot and then watch the colour of your urine. If it turns red, there is not enough hydrochloric acid to break down the colouring in the beetroot. This means it would be helpful to take some hydrochloric acid supplements for a while—but it's better to help your stomach make its own acid by taking herbal bitters and specific nutrients like Vitamin B6, zinc and histidine. Ask your nutritionist. If your urine remains yellow, you are making adequate levels of stomach acid so changing your diet in accordance with Appendix M (or possibly Appendix E—the anti-candida diet) will almost certainly bring relief from indigestion.
- **Empty your bowel at least once every day, *easily!*** You shouldn't need extra bran if you are eating a wholefood diet which is full of fibre but, if you do still suffer from constipation, try adding linseeds to your food, increase your intake of Vitamin C, drink plenty of water and take regular exercise.
- **Take activated charcoal supplements for relief from wind and bloating**—but they won't cure the root cause. Investigate the possibility of candida (see Appendix C—

Candida Score Sheet) and of food allergies (see 'For Action',
Chapter 9).

- **Give thanks to God before eating.** This brief pause will
calm down your overactive mind and body before you try to
digest your food, and will also allow time for the appetising
smells from the kitchen to get your gastric juices flowing
ready to tackle the meal ahead—because that is just what
happens!

CHAPTER 14

AWFUL ACHES—MUSCLE AND JOINT PAIN

'He feels but the pain of his own body' (Job 14:22).

It took me some time to realise that the names of some of our most common complaints have changed. For instance, I discovered that rheumatism is the old-fashioned name for arthritis. You find that it is usually older people who refer to 'rheumatism' in their knees, whereas those who are more up-to-date with current terminology discuss their 'osteoarthritis'. The hospital consultant who specialises in arthritis is still known as a rheumatologist, and 'rheumatism' may still be used for generalised inflammation when it affects both joints and muscles, but basically it is a term which has now been superseded.

Another new word seemed to crop up quite suddenly. I started to hear of many people being diagnosed with fibromyalgia, and I thought it must be some new disease that had just been discovered. Later, I learned that this is the modern name for fibrositis—from which I suffered myself for most of my life.

Regardless of what they might be called, these painful conditions cause a great deal of suffering, sleeplessness and despair. Let's have a look at some of them.

Fibromyalgia is pain in muscle tissue, whereas arthritis affects the joints. It is thought to be caused by improper energy production in the muscles, and it is often helped by taking good levels of magnesium and also of malic acid, from apples. Stress is a major factor in fibromyalgia, because it burns up magnesium in the body. It might be the initial trigger, but equally it might be a virus or a toxic overload.

Besides muscle pain, there is often a collection of other symptoms including fatigue, poor memory and concentration, tingling in hands and feet, headaches, irritability, depression and symptoms of irritable bowel. In this respect, it is very similar to chronic fatigue syndrome, or ME, and in fact some researchers suggest that ME is a continuation from fibromyalgia along the same disease path. As with ME, various possible factors should be suspected, including food allergy, adrenal exhaustion, nutritional deficiencies and candida overgrowth.

Polymyalgia is different in ways which make little difference to the sufferer. Often it is brought on by an over-load of toxins in the body, so it is important to give nutritional support to the liver. As seen in Chapter 10, a common cause of toxins in the body is candida, which releases seventy-nine poisonous substances all the time it is active, so it is not surprising that people suffering from an overgrowth of candida experience a great deal of muscle pain.

Denise had been diagnosed with polymyalgia and she had to resort to regular steroid injections in order to have any freedom from pain and be able to sleep. After just a few months on an anti-candida regime with natural anti-inflammatory and malic acid supplements, together with a good nutritional programme providing plenty of magnesium, she was free of pain and no longer needed the help of steroids.

The two most common types of arthritis are osteoarthritis

and rheumatoid arthritis but it also comes in other forms. Ankylosing spondylitis is a type of arthritis which starts as inflammation of the ligaments but can lead to the fusing-together of vertebrae at the base of the spine and can also spread to other joints.

Gout is actually a form of arthritis and it is fairly commonly experienced as pain and inflammation in the big toe, but it can also affect other joints. It is caused by a build-up of crystals from excess uric acid in the blood, which is normally excreted by the kidneys. Certain types of protein, high in purines, are best avoided in order to reduce the level of uric acid. Purines are high in red meat, liver and kidneys, many seafoods (including mussels, anchovies, sardines), some fish (mackerel, herrings, scallops, sardines) and oats. Very low purine foods include rice, millet, goat's milk and cheese, cottage cheese, green vegetables, nuts, corn and eggs. A high fluid intake is essential to cleanse the system of uric acid, and certain herbal products are helpful to take, especially celery seeds.

Osteoporosis is a loss of bone density, so it is more a disease of the bones than of the joints. It happens most commonly after the menopause, when brittle bones in some cases predispose to multiple fractures. Either insufficient calcium is being deposited in the bones or else too much is being removed. Many situations might be responsible for this, including reduced oestrogen output after the menopause. In addition, an inefficient thyroid gland will not be able to organise the uptake of calcium between blood and bones. Lack of load-bearing exercise also plays a part, as does too much tea or coffee, both of which are responsible for leaching minerals out of the body. It needs a very careful nutritional programme to reverse bone-loss, but bone is living tissue so the situation is by no means hopeless.

Sometimes arthritis is given as a vague diagnosis because it appears to be none of the common types and yet there is still a severe degree of joint pain. Sarah came to me, having suffered with multiple joint pain for several years. Hospital tests had been exhausted, and she had also spent a great deal of money in private clinics to no avail. Blood tests for rheumatoid arthritis were negative and X-rays showed none of the characteristic wear and tear which occurs in osteoarthritis. Having read through previous chapters, perhaps you will not be surprised to learn that I suspected candida, an overgrowth of yeast which would have started in her intestines but migrated elsewhere so that its toxins were causing inflammation in Sarah's joints. In view of the fact that all other tests had proved negative, I put her on an anti-candida regime.

Over the next few weeks it took all my resources to keep her motivated and encouraged because the pains grew steadily worse. Many times she rang me on the point of giving up and stopping the anti-candida diet, but I managed to persuade her to persevere because the increased pain was a sure sign that candida was being destroyed and releasing its toxins in the very places where it had formerly taken up residence, in other words—die-off reaction. Sure enough, after ten weeks Sarah was completely free of joint pain!

Rheumatoid arthritis is a very definite condition, fairly commonly diagnosed by a blood test showing increased levels of rheumatoid factor antibodies. There is no known cure for it, but I have certainly seen its symptoms diminish until they have become virtually non-existent.

We met Bill and his wife on a MasterSun Christian holiday and we become good friends. When Bill learned about our work in nutritional therapy, he asked if anything could be done for rheumatoid arthritis, from which he had been suffering for the past eleven years, mainly affecting his hands, wrists and elbows. It was kept fairly well under control by non-steroidal anti-inflammatory drugs and by monthly injections of a drug derived from gold. His energy levels were not too good, and he had some problems with his skin, especially on his face. He admitted to a strong liking for tea, of which he drank many mugs each day!

I knew that the non-steroidal anti-inflammatory drugs (NSAIDs) would have been causing problems in his digestive tract by destroying friendly bacteria and this, together with factors in his diet including the stimulants in tea, made it pretty certain that he had a candida problem. This would compound the rheumatoid arthritis, first because of the way in which candida seems to make a bee-line for any traumatised tissue and secondly because its toxins cause inflammation. Candida also strongly predisposes to food intolerances, which are frequently found to play a considerable part in rheumatoid arthritis.

The gold-based injections were likely to have had some adverse effects as well, because they can lead to such diverse reactions as rashes, itching, mouth ulcers, diarrhoea, stomach pain, shortness of breath and jaundice. Some of these already appeared on Bill's own list of symptoms.

I urged him to start on the anti-candida diet which, apart from anything else, meant giving up his beloved mugs of tea! The supplements I recommended for him included good levels of GLA (Gamma Linolenic Acid—the active ingredient of borage and evening primrose oil) for its anti-inflammatory properties, and I also advised him to eat plenty of oily fish in order to obtain good levels of EPA, another essential fatty acid with anti-inflammatory properties.

Bill experienced a considerable amount of die-off reaction as candida was destroyed, both in his tummy and in his joints. Everything seemed to get worse, but after three months he reported that a blood test had shown his ESR (erythrocyte sedimentation rate—a measurement of disease and inflammation) had fallen. Three months after that, he wrote to tell me that he no longer needed to take any NSAIDs and had stopped having gold injections. There was still a degree of stiffness in his wrists, but then his nutritional programme still had a way to go so this was not surprising. It was the first time I had experienced someone becoming sufficiently free of the pain of rheumatoid arthritis that a doctor had agreed to stop all types of prescribed medication.

Rheumatoid arthritis is less common than osteoarthritis and it can often affect younger people. It seems to be associated with diet and lifestyle factors, as well as with a faulty immune system, and it can appear quite suddenly, possibly triggered by hereditary factors or by an infection. It starts with inflammation of the membrane which holds the fluid needed to cushion and lubricate the joint. The whole joint then becomes inflamed and enlarged, making movement stiff and painful. A degenerative process is triggered in the cartilage and ultimately in the bone itself, so that the joint becomes mis-shapen. Rheumatoid joints are often warm and the sufferer can run a slight temperature and feel tired and generally run down.

One of the main characteristics is that it attacks symmetrical joints, so that both ankles, both knees or both wrists are affected at the same time. It is an auto-immune disease, which means that your immune system has gone haywire and produces antibodies which attack you instead of attacking an invader. Almost all sufferers have food and chemical sensitivities which encourage a flare-up of symptoms. In tests, grains have been shown to be some of the most common culprits, with wheat or corn affecting more than 50% of sufferers.

Almost as many are affected by gluten grains, which are oats, rye and barley, as well as wheat. Other common allergens include the nightshade family (potatoes, tomatoes, peppers and aubergines), citrus fruits and dairy produce.

Osteoarthritis is the most common type of arthritis. It is a 'wear and tear' disease and so is often accepted as being inevitable, a part of the ageing process, but there is no real reason why this should be the case. It has much more to do with bad posture or injury or over-use or overweight, and it also has to do with eating habits and the biochemical effects of the food we have put into our bodies over the course of a lifetime.

The main symptoms are stiffness and aching, with painful joints which creak. It starts gradually and usually affects just one point at a time, quite often a finger, a knee or a hip (as indicated by the incredible number of people having hip transplants every year). The joints get bigger and the cartilage between the bones degenerates, leading eventually to the formation of bony spurs. There is a loss of flexibility and strength in the joint, as well as varying degrees of pain.

Although osteo- and rheumatoid arthritis are different diseases, they have enough in common to indicate that their treatment may be similar in many respects. The normal medical procedure of giving aspirin and NSAIDs can lead to side-effects and even to a worsening of the disease. For instance, one side-effect of aspirin is that it inhibits the manufacture of connective tissue and this accelerates the breakdown of cartilage. NSAIDs are known to wipe out whole colonies of friendly bacteria in the intestines and to cause ulcers and a 'leaky gut', thus paving the way for more food sensitivities. Like aspirin, they also inhibit collagen and speed up the breakdown of cartilage and, in so doing, encourage arthritis even further. Essential fatty acids like those in evening primrose oil, fish oil and various seeds (sunflower, pumpkin, sesame and flax, also known as linseeds) are at least as effective as NSAIDs or aspirin at reducing inflammation but without side-effects or a risk of accelerating the disease.

When I was in my thirties, I began to experience really severe headaches. Because I had always suffered from sinus problems, I thought that this was the reason once again, but this time the pain was worse than usual. It seemed to radiate from my forehead right over the top of my head, down the back of it and into my neck. Sometimes the pain was so bad that I can remember lying on the floor, pushing my head down against the carpet to try to get some relief, even when I had taken painkillers. I felt the need to keep my head warm, so even indoors I wore a woolly hat and I didn't go out for weeks.

The doctor arranged for my sinuses to be X-rayed but I was told that there seemed to be nothing wrong with them. What the X-rays did show, to my amazement, was osteoarthritis in my neck. I didn't know whether to be relieved about my sinuses or dismayed at the thought of having osteoarthritis when I was still quite young. It came as quite a shock. I realised I had misinterpreted the pattern of the pain; it had not been radiating from the front of my head to the back but the other way round!

An appointment was made for me to see the rheumatologist and he confirmed what the radiographer had said. I asked what could be done about the arthritis and he replied, 'Oh, you'll just have to take painkillers for the rest of your life.' Now I really was dismayed.

Within a few days, I remembered that many years previously, soon after we were married, I had received tremendous help for my damaged back from an osteopath in

London. After five years of severe pain, he was the first one to discover exactly what was wrong. I had seen specialists in three different hospitals, yet no one had found a cause and the only advice I'd been given was to lie on a board when the pain was really bad. This I had done repeatedly, sometimes for weeks on end, beginning to believe that I would spend the rest of my life as an invalid. The relief of hearing the osteopath explain what was wrong was enormous.

He had manipulated my spine and taught me some exercises and it had made an incredible difference. Not surprisingly, I had placed a great deal of confidence in this gentle Swedish osteopath. I suddenly wondered whether, more than ten years on, I could possibly find him again and whether he might be able to do something about my neck and relieve me of some of the terrible pain in my head. I didn't know if he was still in practice—or even if he was still alive. In fact, he was both, and although he had moved, I managed to trace him.

I was delighted that he remembered me from all those years ago, and he was very interested to learn that I had managed to carry and give birth to three babies without reactivating the back problem, though I had to confess to an occasional painful reminder when I neglected to do the exercises! He examined my neck, manipulated and stretched it—and I travelled home from London free of pain for the first time in weeks. I had six sessions with him over three weeks, and it was not until I was getting off the treatment couch for the last time that I noticed a small icon on the wall above it, a picture of Jesus. I knew then that Jesus had been with me all the time and that he had guided the hands of my skilful osteopath. The threatened lifetime of painkillers had been shortened to just a few weeks; now they were no longer needed.

Of course, all this happened long before I was a nutritionist and while I was still eating a great deal of rubbishy food. There is an interesting sequel to the story. Quite recently, my neck was feeling stiff and I thought it would be sensible to ask an osteopath to check it out. This time I saw a young man locally and he carefully examined my neck and my back. He agreed that my neck had stiffened up but said the problem was not in the joints but in the muscles. He also said there seemed to be very little sign of osteoarthritis and, if I hadn't told him, he would not even have suspected that I had been diagnosed as having an osteoarthritic neck more than twenty-five years before.

Even though I left it late in life to change to healthy eating habits and learn about the benefits of vitamins and minerals, the osteoarthritis which had been so severe in my thirties had become a non-event by the time I reached my sixties—yet statistics show that by the age of sixty, over 90% of people show X-ray evidence of arthritic joint-damage. Once again I had found that it is never too late to reap the benefits of nutrition as God intended!

Wise (and Encouraging!) Words

'So here I am today, eighty-five years old! I am still as strong today as the day Moses sent me out; I'm just as vigorous to go out to battle now as I was then'
(Joshua 14:10b–11).

For Action
- **Study carefully Appendix 1 Understanding Arthritis.**
- **Read carefully Chapters 9, 10 and 17,** because inflammation is caused by many things, including food allergies and toxins in the bloodstream.
- **Eat plenty of oily fish and grind up a mixture of**

seeds—sunflower, pumpkin, sesame and linseed (flax)—to add to your cereal or yoghurt. These are full of essential fatty acids which reduce inflammation in the body.

- **Avoid animal fats and red meat**—both will increase inflammation.
- **Avoid fried foods** (including crisps) but if you must fry, use only extra-virgin olive oil.
- **Have a daily salad dressing of good quality sunflower or linseed (flax) oil.**
- **Eat a good, wholefood diet with plenty of fibre** (see Appendix J—Diet for Arthritis), and cut down on (or preferably cut out completely!) sugar and stimulants.
- **Flavour your food with turmeric** for its anti-inflammatory properties.
- **Take a good multivitamin/mineral supplement with extra Vitamin B3 and B5** (each up to 500mg daily) and with good levels of antioxidants such as Vitamins A, C and E and the mineral selenium. (NB Vitamin B3 (niacin) might cause a temporary 'flush', but this is beneficial. If too unpleasant, reduce the level.)
- **Take a magnesium supplement in the form of magnesium malate, and an equal or slightly lower amount of a well-absorbed form of calcium, eg calcium citrate.**
- **Try taking a supplement with Boswellic acid or Glucosamine sulphate,** both of which have natural anti-inflammatory properties.
- **Do all you can to avoid taking pharmaceutical painkillers.** Steroids make your body dependent on them because you stop making your own, and non-steroidal anti-inflammatory drugs (NSAIDs) have a devastating effect on your digestive tract (they are responsible for more drug-related deaths than any other pharmaceutical medication)

while doing nothing about the root cause of the inflammation.

- **Let God handle the stress or anxieties in your life.** Stress increases the production of the adrenal hormone cortisol, which in turn increases inflammation. (See Chapters 7 and 18.)

CHAPTER 15

STARVING AND BINGEING—EATING DISORDERS

'My only food is sighs' (Job 3:24, *Jerusalem Bible*).

'You will eat, but not be satisfied' (Micah 6:14).

I first came across an eating disorder when I was a teenager at school. At the age of fifteen I had been on a music-making holiday with a girl called Alison, both of us with our cellos, and I had got to know her quite well. She was a girl I admired very much—fit and active with a glowing complexion, not really overweight but what would once have been called 'bonny', perhaps carrying just a little puppy-fat. We were not in the same form at school and so our paths did not cross very much, but after a while I realised that I had not seen her around for some time. The word 'anorexia' was rumoured, but I had no idea what it meant. This was in 1950.

After some time, Alison returned to school—and my reaction mirrored that of everyone else when they first saw her. She was thin and gaunt, with bones showing under her skin. Without exaggeration, she was a shadow of her former self. I don't remember how long she stayed at school and I never knew what happened to her, but I well remember the shock of seeing the transformation which had taken place, and I could not begin to imagine why she had decided to starve herself in such a way.

My next encounter with Anorexia nervosa was not for forty years when, as a recently-qualified nutritionist, I was approached by the mother of sixteen-year-old Elizabeth, who had been bed-ridden with ME for three long years. I arranged to visit them and found this girl lying immobile in a darkened room, looking painfully thin and pale. Her mother said that Elizabeth could eat only a very few foods because there were so many to which she reacted very severely. Of those she did eat, she would have no more than a spoonful or two.

Something in me rang warning bells. Although I have many clients who do indeed suffer from multiple food sensitivities, I somehow suspected that Elizabeth might be manipulating her situation by telling her mother that everything she ate just made her feel worse, which actually meant that she was very strictly controlling the amount of food which went into her body. Each day she was fed just a few spoonfuls of food, and each day she just lay in her bed, getting thinner and thinner. My suspicions of anorexia were confirmed when Elizabeth's mother told me that her daughter would sometimes look down at her skinny body as she lay on the bed, and say, 'Look at me, I'm so fat!'

One day, Elizabeth's mother rang me in great distress because the doctor had said that if Elizabeth did not gain some weight in the following week, he would have to put her in hospital so that she could be given a glucose drip. This worried both mother and daughter because they now understood that an overgrowth of the yeast, *Candida albicans*, was probably playing a large part in Elizabeth's ME, and they knew that glucose would simply 'feed' the yeast in her body. She asked if there was anything I could possibly do in so short a time to try to avoid the hospital and the glucose drip.

I had learned that specific amino acid supplements could sometimes work wonders with eating disorders by providing much-needed protein in a way which can be easily absorbed and restore the biochemical balance in the body and also in the mind. I said I would provide some suitable supplements and, if Elizabeth really was more anxious to avoid going to hospital than she was of possibly gaining some weight, I would expect her to co-operate with me by taking a very high level of the amino acid supplements, as many as fifteen capsules every day. Elizabeth agreed.

Just five days later, the tide had turned. Elizabeth lay on her bed and looked at her body and said, 'Look at me, Mummy, I'm all skin and bone. Please will you bring me something to eat?' The first miracle had happened; Elizabeth's distorted self-perception had been corrected by taking the nutrients which her brain had been lacking, some simplé amino acids. They went on to encourage the stimulation of her gastric juices, thereby improving her appetite, and it wasn't long before Elizabeth's body started to work well in other ways, including hormonally. After a while, the Lord allowed her to be completely healed of her chronic fatigue syndrome through loving prayer ministry.

Eating disorders are not just confined to young girls, but Alison's story and Elizabeth's are fairly typical. What was not typical was the speed with which Elizabeth overcame the anorexia, which frequently takes months or even years of patient counselling.

Another type of eating disorder is Bulimia nervosa, when sufferers are caught up in a cycle of binge and vomit (or binge and purge). Often they appear to eat normally but then make themselves sick in order to control their weight. Sometimes they take laxatives or diuretics for the same reason, and sometimes they become exercise addicts because they are so fearful of putting on weight.

When I was training as a nutritionist, I had to set up a research project and I chose to research the effects of amino acids on eating disorders. I wrote an article for our local paper, requesting volunteers. Anorexics and bulimics are normally secretive about their condition but, even so, twenty volunteers enrolled for the project. Pamela told me that as soon as she read the article, she said to herself, 'Enough is enough!' She had been bulimic for thirty years, since the age of twelve—and no one had ever suspected, not even her husband. After every meal, she simply took herself to the toilet and made herself sick. In this way, she appeared to be eating normally but kept a tight rein on her weight.

Not surprisingly, she had become ill in various ways because she had absorbed so few nutrients over so many years. I recommended that she take the amino acid supplements for a full three months, and I also provided some optional dietary guidelines if she wanted to use them. Basically, I wanted to take the emphasis in her thinking away from food and simply let the amino acids do their work.

After just ten weeks, Pamela was totally free of bulimia and was feeling very well. In fact, she had opted to follow the diet guidelines so she had received a double benefit. At the end of the first week, this is what she wrote: 'After I came to see you, I made the momentous decision to tell my husband the whole story. I think he was quite shocked, but he has been really supportive and we talked for a long time. I would like to thank you for being the catalyst that resulted in my telling my husband about my eating disorder.' After sixteen weeks, at the end of the research project, she wrote: 'Thank you for all you've done—not least the new lease of life you've given me.'

Eating disorders usually fall into one of three types:

1. Compulsive over-eating, when the sufferer constantly goes on diets but gains the weight back in between, suffering extreme feelings of guilt and remorse.

2. Anorexia, when food intake is strictly limited and controlled, causing extreme underweight but a distorted view of their own body image.

3. Bulimia, involving secret purging after apparently normal eating but also frequently characterised by binges followed by purges.

However, there is a lot of overlap between these three conditions. It has been reported that about one in two hundred girls in the age group fifteen to eighteen suffers from an eating disorder, but it is also quite common in older age groups. The incidence in men is on the increase due to a preoccupation with lean, athletic appearance, and it is a worrying fact that the number of children affected is also growing.

Eating disorders give rise to physical and mental side-effects which can sometimes prove tragically fatal, and the suffering extends to the whole family, whose own lives can be ruled by the illness and who often feel guilty and responsible for the situation.

A lot of emphasis has been put on the psychological aspect of these illnesses, but as a nutritionist I have become increasingly convinced of the role played by various physical conditions, with possibly a psychological trigger being the spark which lights the fire. For instance, as already seen, nutritional deficiencies can play a part in anorexia so that neither the body nor the brain is able to work properly and then, of course, a vicious circle is established. Sometimes just a throw-away comment about a girl's size or shape is the trigger which will make her embark on a diet so extreme that she loses all control of it.

One explanation is that, if we are lacking in zinc, we do not have an appetite, so if a girl has previously been a 'picky eater' and her diet has provided little or no zinc (found in red meat, fish, seafood, pumpkin seeds, eggs, nuts and whole grains), her appetite will already be poor. Added to this, zinc is used for the growth of every cell in the body, so copious amounts are needed in puberty. The root cause of a teenage girl's eating disorder is often therefore a simple nutritional deficiency of zinc which was already in existence before a possible thoughtless remark made her desperately want to get slim, or her parents' divorce made her want to create some control in her life. It was then easy to stop eating because she had no appetite, anyway—and the less she ate, the less zinc went into her body so that all traces of appetite totally disappeared. And a zinc-deficiency is a situation which no amount of counselling will cure!

Compulsive eating and uncontrollable binges have several possible physical explanations, the first of which is food allergy or intolerance. If we have an intolerance to a certain food without realising (the effect becomes 'masked' or hidden if we eat it on a regular basis) and therefore continue to eat it, the immune system is affected in such a way that we actually end up addicted to that food. Katy was a beautiful seventeen-year-old girl who volunteered for my research project. She suffered so severely from bulimia that her mother had to put padlocks on every cupboard door in the kitchen and on the fridge and freezer. One night, however, she had forgotten to put away all the shopping and she left a bag of flour on the table. In the middle of the night, Katy went downstairs and ate her way through a whole bag of raw flour. We learned from this experience that she was heavily addicted to wheat, and its hold on her was as powerful as heroin!

Another situation which might trigger an episode of bingeing is when blood sugar levels are low and trigger symptoms of fatigue, anxiety, etc., which we feel we must fight off by eating lots of sweet foods (see Chapter 8). Yet another trigger is yeast infection, or candidiasis, when the presence of an overgrowth of yeast causes cravings for the foods it requires in order to thrive (see Chapter 10).

You might not think that it is possible for a modern-day Westerner to suffer from malnutrition, but in fact the standard Western diet consists mainly of empty calories, food which is filling but lacking in nutrients, and this can cause a significant increase in appetite. When the liver becomes depleted of essential nutrients, it reacts by sending hunger signals to the brain. This might be yet another way in which a binge is triggered.

Alcohol, drugs and even several medications (antihistamines, antidepressants and tranquillisers) are all known to stimulate appetite, often leading in young people to a marked increase in food intake and in some cases encouraging a latent addictive tendency.

With this and other information in mind, I was eager to see what might be achieved by my research project. Thirteen of the eighteen who completed the trial responded to some extent to nutritional supplementation with amino acids, and some of them did extremely well, including Pamela. Of the few who did not respond, it was fairly evident that there were still physical as well as psychological components to their problems but I was not able to tackle these within the limitations of the trial. However, sufficient improvement was seen overall to confirm that neither the mind nor the body can work efficiently when they are under-fuelled with amino acids and other nutrients. Amino acids have been shown to supply the best possible fuel in the quickest way to ensure the repair and then the efficient working of all the cells in the body.

Although the earliest written account of anorexia appears as far back as 1689 and the first medical accounts were published in 1873, eating disorders have risen alarmingly in the years since 1950. The psychological reasons for this increase must surely include a desire to conform to the media image of apparently-starved young women who personify the current view of beauty. In addition, there are the fears and anxieties which develop as a result of increasingly common family breakdown. The scene for an eating disorder is set when you add to these, and countless other emotional stresses, the fact that our modern-day diet consists mainly of empty calories, providing very little fuel for our physical and mental machinery.

Thank God that for many sufferers, struggling with guilt, self-disgust and low self-esteem as well as with all the physical effects of self-induced starvation, there are in fact some answers. First, there is the love and wisdom of God available through Christians, and then there is the responsible application of nutritional therapy.

If you yourself have an eating disorder, determine now to bring it to God for the very last time and then look to him expectantly for answers and trust him to lead you to the help which you require. I am convinced that he not only longs to set you free but that he will really do it. Why else do you find yourself reading these words?

Wise Words

'Now the Lord is the Spirit, and where the Spirit of the Lord is, there is freedom' (2 Corinthians 3:13).

'But the fruit of the Spirit is . . . self-control. Those who belong to Christ Jesus have crucified the sinful nature with its passions and desires. Since we live by the Spirit, let us keep in step with the Spirit' (Galatians 5:22, 24–25).

For Action

- **Determine to be honest with yourself.** Are you making excuses for not eating? Or for always eating too much, or for taking diuretics or laxatives, or for being an exercise fanatic?

- **If you know in your heart that you are anorexic,** acknowledge that the enemy is trying to rob you of your health—and of your life—by starving you to death. Give your life anew to Jesus and determine to be whole. Show you mean it by taking a good zinc supplement (eg Zinc Citrate 15mg × 2 daily) as a first step towards increasing your interest in food, and a good amino acid complex to correct the imbalances in your body and your mind.

- **If you know in your heart that you are bulimic,** try to find a physical reason for your cravings and binges so that you no longer need to feel guilty about your weak will-power. (See Chapters 8, 9 and 10.)

- **Determine to be honest with other people** about your problem, and ask for help—both spiritual and nutritional.

- **Determine to be honest with God,** and read again the last paragraph of this chapter and the 'Wise Words' from Scripture which follow it.

CHAPTER 16

UNHAPPY HORMONES—SEXUAL CHEMISTRY

'Do not look angry, my lord, because I cannot stand in your presence, for I am as women are from time to time' (Genesis 31:35, *Jerusalem Bible*).

Let me start this chapter with tales of two young women, both in their early thirties and both of them Christians. The first, Ellen, very much wanted a baby but had suffered the emotional and physical trauma of no less than five miscarriages. When she came to see me, she had also been suffering from ME for some time, so life was not too happy for her.

Hospital investigations had shown that Ellen had very low levels of progesterone, and since this is the hormone needed to 'hold' a newly fertilised egg in place until the placenta is strong enough to take over, low progesterone was evidently the reason for her many failed pregnancies. Ellen was offered progesterone treatment but she really did not want to take it; she decided she would much rather see whether her hormone levels could be regulated by nutritional means.

And they were! By the time she had taken nutritional supplements to improve her overall health and had also brought candida overgrowths under control, Ellen's progesterone levels were so good that, when she conceived another baby, she was able to carry it throughout the pregnancy and eventually gave birth to a bouncing baby boy. No form of 'hormone therapy' had been necessary.

Laura was a district nurse. She had been married for several years and had come to terms with the fact that she would never be able to have a baby because she had not had a period since the age of twenty-one and, after thorough medical investigations, she had been told that her ovaries had atrophied. Laura and her husband were in the process of adopting beautiful twin baby girls, so she had dealt with the grief of her infertility and was busy building a positive future. However, she was keen to have a good nutritional programme worked out for her so that she could be in the best possible health.

Both Laura and I were amazed when, after four months on the programme, she had a period—the first in eleven years! That is not to say that her reproductive system was fully functioning, but it was incredible to see that optimum nutrition could make such a difference to atrophied ovaries that they suddenly regained sufficient function to trigger a menstrual flow.

These two stories show something of what can happen when we take steps to co-operate with the body by providing it with all the nutrients it needs to work efficiently—and to heal itself. Controversy rages about hormone therapy, and I'll come to that later, but these two case studies show that there really is a viable alternative in the form of nutritional therapy, although unfortunately it is realised by all-too-few people and most women believe that they have no choice other than some form of hormone treatment.

Some women are also under the mistaken impression that the hormone therapy prescribed by their doctor is not synthetic but is natural, and so is perfectly safe to use.

Unfortunately, there is not much that is natural to the female body about hormones which have been extracted from the urine of pregnant mares and then chemically adapted to make them fit for human use! Admittedly, they were natural to female horses originally, but they no longer form a natural substance once they have been pharmaceutically developed—and they are certainly not natural to the human female body!

Let's think about some of the problems which can be caused by inefficient or irregular hormone function. First, there can be problems at puberty; periods can start when a girl is so young that she finds it difficult to cope with them emotionally and physically, or they can start very late so that she is worried because all her friends have periods and she does not. Periods can be embarrassingly heavy with severe pain, and there can be erratic emotions and behaviour or painful, swollen breasts for several days beforehand. Then there are problems in pregnancy, or problems of infertility, and eventually there are problems in the menopausal years—hot flushes, night sweats, insomnia, depression, anxiety and irritability which, combined with a fear of developing osteoporosis, lead an increasing number of doctors to prescribe hormone replacement therapy (HRT).

Any or all of these problems are accepted by most women as being part of life, part of what it means to be a woman, and some Christian women believe strongly that these are problems which God allows us to bear in order to give us the opportunity to draw more of our strength from him. That may well be true, but he also provides answers so that we don't need to have these problems in the first place. An optimally-nourished body is much less likely to experience premenstrual, menstrual or menopausal symptoms, and an optimally-nourished mother has a far greater chance of a problem-free pregnancy with a healthy baby at the end of it.

Levels of hormones are constantly changing in menstruating women and they have an amazingly powerful effect both on our bodies and our minds, but we need to realise that we do not have to succumb to their power or be controlled by them. After all, hormones are made from components of the food which we eat, so it stands to reason that if we eat the right sort of food, we shall be in control of our hormonal function and not the other way around. This applies to all the hormones in our body, whether thyroxine from the thyroid gland, insulin from the pancreas, adrenaline, cortisol and DHEA from the adrenal glands or oestrogen and progesterone from the ovaries. If we provide the right sort of building materials in the right sort of balance, our hormones will also be balanced.

The contraceptive pill and HRT are both types of synthetic hormones and, as they have to be as much like our own hormones as possible, they enter the body as fatty steroids. The problem with putting steroids into the body is that our glands learn to rely on them and we stop making our own. Apart from anything else, this has the effect of weakening the immune system, a situation which is sometimes extremely difficult to reverse even when steroid treatments are stopped, and it leaves our own sex hormone function even more irregular than it was before. It takes many months for the hormone cycle to become normal when the Pill is stopped.

The first line of defence in the immune system is made up of secretory antibodies which create a barrier on the intestinal wall, and this is very often the first area to suffer when, for instance, a woman has been on the Pill for some time. Disturbed antibodies on the intestinal lining encourage an imbalance of microbes, and the most opportunistic of the 'bad guys', *Candida albicans*, is then encouraged to overgrow.

The Pill is one of the main causes of yeast infection, and HRT is just as bad.

Since weakened immunity and an overgrowth of candida both figure largely in cases of chronic fatigue syndrome, or ME, any type of hormonal intervention is one of the main culprits we look for when trying to discover how the illness might have gained a hold. The media carry reports of famous women who sing the praises of HRT but my reaction is to sit back and wait to see how their health is faring in a few years' time. There are in fact quite a few potential side-effects and risks attached to HRT, besides the fact that it weakens immunity, thereby encouraging yeast infection and other effects of a compromised immune system. The side-effects include depression, high blood pressure (therefore an increased risk of blood clots, strokes and heart disease), phlebitis (inflammation of a vein) and an increased risk of cancer of the womb and breast. It is reckoned to take seven years for HRT to provide protection against osteoporosis and researchers have found that even those women who stayed on HRT for ten years experienced a rapid decline in bone density when they eventually stopped taking it, so that by the age of seventy-five their bone mass was only 3.2% higher than in women who had never taken HRT. It there-fore seems reasonable to ask whether the potential risks are worth taking, especially since there is a completely safe alter-native approach which is easily accessible. A combination of healthy foods, vitamin and mineral supplements and regular weight-bearing exercise (such as walking) is known to help protect against osteoporosis.

When Janet arrived at my door, I described her afterwards as 'a puddle on the doorstep'. She was a pretty woman, but she was crying uncontrollably and she looked ill and woe-begone. She was in her early forties, though she looked much younger. She had no children but she had been recommended to have a hysterectomy to put an end to her period problems. After the operation, she was put on HRT. When she became ill and depressed, her consultant said that she obviously needed a stronger dose of HRT, which he administered as an implant. The effect of this was to make her so depressed that she was almost suicidal, and she was absolutely desperate for help when she found me.

I soon realised that the steroid effect of the HRT had encouraged a tremendous overgrowth of candida, which in turn was releasing all its toxins and these were poisoning her body and her brain, quite literally. The problem was that the implant would continue to release its steroids into Janet's body for six more months.

She decided to spend a lot of money in asking her gynaecologist to remove the implant, but when he attempted to do so he found that it had disintegrated and dispersed throughout her body. Somehow I found ways of encouraging and 'nursing' her through the following months, all the time trying to prevent the candida overgrowth from getting further out of control. Eventually, the time came when the effects of the patch wore off, the nutritional programme kicked in and candida came under control—and then I was able to meet the real Janet, who has a delightful *joie de vivre* and is the last person you would think could ever become depressed. I still see her frequently and she remains a great enthusiast for optimum nutrition. Not surprisingly, she is now one of the most 'anti-HRT' people I know!

Many women are aware of the dangers of HRT and so they jumped at the possibility of a natural alternative when it appeared on the scene—so-called 'natural' progesterone cream. This is a controversial substance over which reputable nutritionists come down firmly on differing sides of the fence. My own view is that by the time you apply the cream there is nothing natural about it because it has been chemically modified into something quite different from its original state when it was extracted from a wild yam or soya bean.

Those who favour natural progesterone treatment explain that it regulates a state of oestrogen-dominance, which is responsible for most types of menopausal problems and also for PMS, ovarian cysts, breast lumps, fibroids, infertility, miscarriage and even more. However, others are not so happy with it because they believe that it is still an artificially-introduced hormonal substance which is just as likely to upset the steroid apple-cart (immunity, hormone function, etc.), as the overtly synthetic variety. It certainly interferes with the feed-back cycle in the glands, in which the hypothalamus in the brain is told by the ovaries to make whichever hormones are needed. All this occurs, and yet women think they are simply taking a simple, harmless herbal remedy. Fortunately, in Britain now, natural progesterone is available only on prescription, but many natural practitioners are encouraging their clients to ask their doctors to prescribe it, or even to send for it from abroad. My personal view is that this should not be necessary if the nutritional status is properly sorted out. If God has decided that our bodies should stop producing progesterone at a certain age, who are we to put it back again?

I have my own story to tell about natural progesterone. A few years ago, well after I had stopped menstruating and when natural progesterone was making its first debut in Britain, I thought I would try the cream to see if it would benefit my skin, vaginal tissues and general well-being as was claimed. (It did not need a prescription at that time.) As advised, I rubbed a little onto the inside of my thighs, from where it would be absorbed into my bloodstream. I started a week before we were due to go on holiday in Corfu. On our fourth day there, we booked to go on a jeep safari into the mountains—and I woke up that morning with horrendous abdominal cramps and bleeding. In lectures and books on natural progesterone, I had learned that for a few months this was likely to happen, as the menstrual cycle is temporarily reactivated in post-menopausal women. It is one thing to hear about and another to experience it after several years of having no periods. On what should have been a care-free day of adventure, I had to endure pain, anxiety and inconvenience—and I vowed that I would never inflict this situation on one of my clients. And I certainly did not intend to put up with it for a few more months while my hormones went through a reshuffle! My 'natural' progesterone cream went straight into the bin.

Of course, if natural progesterone cream is prescribed by a doctor, he has the facility to carry out an examination if there is cause for concern, to reassure or to refer to a gynaecologist if necessary. If it is recommended by a nutritionist, there is no such facility and the client's doctor might justifiably be angry that he has been asked to prescribe a substance which has caused such unacceptable effects.

The original proponent of hormone therapy was a man. My pet theory is that he was wanting a quiet life for himself while his wife went through the menopause! The original proponent of natural progesterone cream is also a man, and I think that if he had to endure what I lived through on that holiday in Corfu, he would possibly be a little less keen to advocate it! I know others who have also had unhappy experiences with natural progesterone cream and I am writing this so that you may realise that possibly it is not quite the best thing since sliced bread (and who said *that* was good?!).

The menopause is not an illness or a disease caused by a

lack of hormones which can therefore be made better by taking more hormones. If there are unpleasant symptoms, this is often due to other reasons such as the effects of a depletion or imbalance of nutrients in the body, or an over-growth of candida which, as explained in Chapter 10, can really mess up hormone function and conversely will have its own symptoms made worse by changes in hormone levels.

In many other cultures, menopausal symptoms are rare; once again, we have created our own Western disease by the food we eat. It is surely better to help the body to sort itself out by giving it the right fuel so that it can make its own adjustments, rather than giving it props (whether synthetic or 'natural') to rely upon. When it comes to adjusting hor-mones, there are many therapeutic herbs to help in this process (eg Agnus Castus, Black Cohosh, Dong Quai), but the essential factor is to correct and improve your nutritional status.

Women are not the only ones with hormones; men have them too! Too much of a hormone called DHT (dihydrotes-tosterone) is what leads to male baldness and benign pros-tate problems. Originally, orthodox medicine attempted to treat prostate problems with drugs which were male hormone-blockers, and later with drugs to deal directly with DHT. In both cases, there were terrible side-effects and these approaches had to be abandoned. Then researchers discov-ered a berry called Saw Palmetto which was astoundingly effective at stopping DHT production, and it is now one of the most widely-prescribed treatments by doctors in Europe, though sadly not yet in Britain.

Women can also be affected by DHT because they produce small amounts of the male hormone testosterone and if there is too much of it, this will lead to the production of DHT which is even more potent. This situation can lead to polycystic ovaries, an overgrowth of facial and bodily hair or hair-loss on the head. Once again, Saw Palmetto can often be extremely helpful, especially in conjunction with the herb Dong Quai and appropriate nutritional supplements to help support the pituitary, ovaries and adrenal glands.

The human reproductive system is one of the great marvels of God's design, and he planned it to bring us joy, first of all in giving men and women the opportunity to share the deepest act of love and then to watch the woman's body swell and eventually to share together the thrill of welcoming a new life into their arms. Even though God says in Genesis that woman shall give birth in pain, how quickly he overshadows that pain with joy when she holds her new baby!

He has certainly not said that women should suffer for half of their lives because of their menstrual cycle, or that they should suffer when that cycle comes to an end. He loves his children and wants them to be in health, women as well as men; able to experience fullness of life just as Jesus promised; to share that health and life and joy with their husbands and children, unhindered by regular weeks of pain and irritability. I believe he wants his daughters, as they grow older and have fewer family ties, not just to await old age in decreasing activity and increasing ill health but to be well and strong to tackle new work for him, reaching out in ways which have been impossible before. We need to reconsider our expectations and rid ourselves of basic misconceptions. God wants us whole. Not just a little bit and not just some of the time, but whole all over and all of the time.

Dozens of times a year I hear from women who, having been following a nutritional programme, are absolutely amazed that for the first time they can remember they have suffered not a single premenstrual symptom. They say they had no indication that a period was on its way until it arrived. I hear from dozens of others that, when they had spent a few weeks improving their nutritional status in ways I had recommended and then had stopped taking HRT, the menopausal symptoms which they dreaded had simply not returned.

Perhaps the biggest joy is hearing from women who have been infertile until their late thirties but have now been able to conceive. A little trouble sorting out your nutrition can have some marvellous consequences.

Hormonal problems such as those commonly experienced at the menopause—hot flushes, heavy perspiration, insomnia, anxiety attacks and so on—only occur because for the whole of our lives we have been putting poor-grade fuel into our body's machinery. Up-grade the fuel, clean out the machine, gently crank up the gears, and our bodies will run as smoothly as they were designed to do; we just didn't know it was possible. But our heavenly Father knows. He made us so that our wheels would run smoothly; how sad he must be to see us all clogged up, slowed down and growing rusty!

Make up your mind that you want to change the situation, and you can be certain that our master designer and engineer will help you get it right.

Wise Words

'She is clothed with strength and dignity; she can laugh at the days to come' (Proverbs 31:25).

For Action

• Several chapters in this book have some bearing on the way your hormones work. **As any situations become clear, follow the advice on what to do**—whether it is improving your nutritional status, supporting your adrenal glands, detoxifying your liver or bringing candida under control.

- **Stop using the Pill**—use an alternative method of contraception or look to good nutrition to help sort out your menstrual problems. The Pill is a form of steroid and over time it will weaken your immunity. The same applies to Hormone Replacement Therapy.
- **Follow a good healthy diet.** (See Appendix M.)
- **Take a good multivitamin/mineral supplement,** or preferably ask a nutritionist to formulate a tailor-made programme of supplements for you.
- **For any hormonal problems, take a high dose of evening primrose oil** or other supplements containing the essential fatty acid GLA.
- **If you suffer from PMT or breast pain, take GLA as above and also capsules of the herb Agnus Castus × 2 daily,** the first as soon as you wake and the other at noon.
- **If you suffer from period pain or irregularities, take GLA as above and supplements of the herb Dong Quái × 3 daily.**
- **If you have menopausal symptoms, eg hot flushes, take the herb Black Cohosh × 1 daily.** It's a good alternative to HRT.
- **Make time for some weight-bearing exercise such as walking** and carrying your shopping. This, together with an appropriate nutritional programme, will guard against osteoporosis.
- **Believe that God wants you free to be well and active,** like the perfect wife in Proverbs 31, so that you, too, can be 'clothed with strength and dignity and laugh at the days to come' (Proverbs 31:25).

CHAPTER 17

OVERLOADED LIVERS—TOXICITY

'My prayer is not that you take them out of the world but that you protect them from the evil one' (John 17:15).

Soon after I had qualified, Samantha consulted me for help with chronic fatigue syndrome. She was a young mother, with one little girl about to start school and a toddler aged eighteen months. She had not been well for some time but had been completely without strength since the birth of the baby. She was a typical candida candidate but she responded only slightly to the initial anti-candida programme, and then reached a plateau because as soon as she tried to take anti-fungal supplements, she became even more ill.

I suspected that her liver was having difficulty coping with high levels of toxins because, even in the absence of any other toxic invaders, candida had been releasing seventy-nine chemical substances into her body all the time it had been in a state of overgrowth. Then, as soon as she started to kill the fungus, it released a great many more toxins—the dreaded candida 'die-off' effect.

I advised her to try a simple herbal supplement containing silymarin, or milk thistle, because this herb has been known for generations for its liver-support properties. Two months later, Samantha telephoned me to say that for the past week or so she had been walking at least half a mile every day to the school and back, and had even been able to push the baby's buggy for the first time since the baby had been born. Samantha still had quite a long way to go before she would be fully well, but there was no doubting the encouragement she felt by having turned a considerable corner.

A few years on, I was contacted by the mother of nine-teen-year-old Julie. Julie was in an even worse state than Samantha, having been in bed with ME for the past two years, almost completely immobile. As sometimes happens in these situations, her hands had contracted into a claw shape. I started her on a good nutritional programme which took account of her very obvious candida overgrowth as well as low blood sugar, hormonal situations and general nutritional deficiencies. As with Samantha, there was a little improvement but basically Julie was still lying in bed with her hands clenched up like little claws.

She started to take very low levels of antifungal supple-ments to destroy the candida overgrowth in her body, but soon she began to feel even worse. I guessed that her liver was not able to cope with the extra load of toxins being released by candida as it was destroyed. I had kept up with post-grad-uate studies and by this time I had learned more about how the body copes with toxins.

Removal of waste material is essential for the healthy working of our bodies, which have many different ways of off-loading it. We get rid of waste products when we per-spire, when we breathe and when we sneeze. In addition, the kidneys filter waste from our blood and excrete it in urine, and our bowels get rid of toxins which have been released in bile from the liver, excreting them together with what is left of our food after we have absorbed its nutrients.

Central to all of this is the role of the liver which, among other things, has the tremendous responsibility of producing many thousands of enzymes, regulating blood sugar, filtering blood, manufacturing bile, breaking down old red blood cells and hormones, producing cholesterol and detoxifying harmful substances. This latter role of detoxification is performed in two stages. Phase I turns the toxins into substances which are even more poisonous than they were to start with! This happens in order to kick-start phase II into operation, which then turns the toxins into safe substances for the kidneys to excrete.

If too many toxins enter the body, phase II has difficulty in keeping up with detoxifying the high level of poisons being thrown at its door by phase I. In this situation, toxins build up, accumulating not only in the liver and kidneys but also in the brain and in fatty tissue throughout the body. No wonder people say they feel ill all over; they are actually being poisoned due to the inefficiency of their own bodies! However, if phase II can be encouraged to work efficiently once more, the toxins will be cleaned out from their various storage sites, and this will lead to improvements in general well-being, both physical and mental. Phase II can in fact be strengthened by providing the liver with all the nutrients it needs, including amino acids, to produce the enzymes necessary for its responsible job of work.

I suggested such a programme of nutrients to Julie's mother, and Julie decided that she would like to give it a try. A few weeks later, I answered my telephone to hear Julie herself on the line.

'Hello!' I said. 'You must be feeling better to be talking on the telephone. This is the first time we've spoken.'

'Yes,' she said. 'And I wanted to tell you that I am sitting downstairs and I'm dressed.'

I was delighted to know that her hands were no longer curled up like claws; another happy client had turned a corner. Julie had been virtually paralysed by the effects of an overworked and exhausted liver.

Quite often, when people start to feel better they begin to move about more and take some gentle exercise. Then, next day, they are disappointed to find that they feel worse again. They ring me up and say, 'I'm having a relapse!', and I hurry to reassure them that this is not in fact the case.

I explain to them that toxins are collected up in the lymphatic system, which is a drainage system running all around our bodies. Unlike the bloodstream, it doesn't have a pump of its own. The pump for the lymphatic system is literally our own physical activity; the movement of our muscles pushes toxins round our bodies until they are tipped into the bloodstream via the thoracic duct at the base of the neck. When toxins are being carried by the lymphatics we don't notice them, but when they are in the bloodstream they make us ache all over and feel generally ill.

You can see from this that a period of extra or unaccustomed activity would be responsible for tipping a whole lot of toxins into the bloodstream all at once, causing you to feel ill all over and poisoned once again, just when you thought you had started to get better. It isn't really a relapse; it just feels like one. If the liver is healthy, this will only be a temporary situation because the blood will be detoxified quickly and efficiently, but an unhealthy liver will be overwhelmed, and the accumulated toxins will continue to circulate in your bloodstream, making you feel ill in a wide variety of ways.

Before considering the possibility that phase II has gone

into a stage of exhaustion (and this can actually be shown by a very helpful diagnostic laboratory test), there are a number of simple steps to try which are often all that needs to be done to help to clean up the liver and improve the efficiency of its detoxification processes. Apart from taking the herb silymarin, as Samantha did, the first essential tip is to drink as much filtered or purified water as you possibly can. This will help to flush the toxins out of your body through the kidneys.

The second tip is to take plenty of Vitamin C, up to what is known as 'bowel tolerance levels'. This simply means that you have taken enough Vitamin C to cause a loose bowel motion. When the body is full of toxins, or equally, when it is fighting an infection or an allergy, it will soak up Vitamin C like a sponge. But when its tissues have reached saturation point, Vitamin C will then be off-loaded via the bowel, causing slight diarrhoea. Vitamin C is the one nutrient for which our requirement varies not only from person to person but also from day to day. Sometimes as little as 1 gram (1,000mg) will cause diarrhoea, but occasionally someone will need to take 30 grams (30,000mg) or even more before experiencing a loose motion.

Vitamin C therefore performs a multiple role in this situation. Besides being a natural antioxidant which neutralises nasty free radical molecules, and also having immune-boosting and antihistamine effects, it detoxifies the tissues and then encourages the elimination of the toxins from the body. It is essential to guard against constipation at all costs, because toxins are absorbed through the bowel lining back into the bloodstream—especially if there is a leaky gut or a low level of antibodies lining the wall—creating an even greater load on the liver. It is actually impossible to stay constipated if you take enough Vitamin C! The next day, once things are moving, you will probably need less to achieve the same result, and so on.

From time to time there are scare-mongering attempts in the media about purported dangers of vitamins, and Vitamin C was one which came under attack. However, the report was no more than an assumption based on incomplete research which did not stand up to scientific scrutiny and so was discounted by nutritionally-informed medical practitioners and by nutritionists. I personally took a minimum of 15 grams (15,000mg) of Vitamin C daily for many years, increasing to considerably more when I was experiencing die-off reaction, infections or allergies, and I am certain that without it I would not now be here to tell the tale!

One other useful tip in a strategy to cleanse the liver is to drink 'coffee' made from dandelion root, either roasted or unroasted. The roasted variety makes a useful alternative to proper coffee and is a really very pleasant drink. Dandelion root has various roles; it stimulates the production of bile which in turn carries toxins out of the liver. Stools tend to look darker when you drink dandelion coffee, due to the increased amount of bile, and you know that the increase in colour also means an increase in the elimination of toxins. In addition, dandelion root is known to medical herbalists as a 'bitter', which means that it aids digestion by stimulating the production of gastric juices. If digestion is poor, it is a good idea to drink a cup of dandelion coffee fifteen minutes before a meal. Another role of dandelion root is as an aperient, which means that it gently encourages an easy bowel movement without having an actual laxative effect.

The fact that it is also a very pleasant drink means that you cannot go very far wrong by drinking plenty of dandelion coffee. Treat it as a normal drink and have half a dozen cups a day. Don't buy dandelion coffee in a jar, especially if you suspect or are fighting a candida problem, because it contains lactose. Instead, buy roasted dandelion root and, if you have any coffee-making equipment, grind the root pieces and then make in the same way as ordinary coffee, using a filter jug, percolator or coffee machine. Otherwise, simply place two heaped teaspoonsful into a saucepan with about nine cups of water (weaker or stronger as preferred), bring to the boil and simmer for fifteen minutes. Heat up a cupful whenever you feel like a drink. Incidentally, this is not to be confused with dandelion tea which is made from the leaves and not the root; these have a useful diuretic effect but are not so effective as a liver tonic.

So what sort of toxins create a load on the liver? Some come from inside our own bodies, like candida toxins and traces of mercury from dental fillings, and others come from outside. Unfortunately, they come at us from all directions—from the earth and the air, from water and from what we put into ourselves in food and drink and also medicines. It's quite a sordid picture.

In 1990, there were 70,000 chemicals in common use in pesticides, foods and drugs, and this number grows by many thousands every year. The average person eats 5kg (12lb) of chemical additives every year, and 4.5 litres (a gallon) of herbicides and pesticides which have been sprayed onto fruit and vegetables.

Lead is a toxic metal which we inhale from exhaust fumes, and which we eat because the traffic fumes have landed on vegetables and grains as they grow in the fields. In addition, cows eat grass which has lead on it so it enters our bodies in milk, cheese and beef. Lead interferes with the behaviour of the brain, causing learning problems, hyperactivity and aggression in children. Cadmium is another toxic metal which we inhale from exhausts and also from smoke, whether from factory chimneys or from cigarettes. Aluminium is now medically acknowledged to play a role in memory loss and in Alzheimer's disease, a form of senile dementia.

Our water supply is high in nitrates because they are used in fertilisers and have filtered through the soil into our rivers and reservoirs, yet some water authorities still do not have the necessary purification equipment. Vegetables and grains are grown with nitrate fertilisers and nitrates are also added to cured meats such as ham and bacon and to sausages and pies. Once inside the body, nitrates combine with other foods to produce highly cancer-producing substances.

The same sort of story can be told about pesticides, which are known to be poisonous, yet some fruits, particularly strawberries, raspberries, grapes and tomatoes, have been found to contain six different pesticides!

The consumption of medical drugs in Britain is reported to be the highest in the world. Residues from any type of medication will build up in the liver, and self-induced liver problems are of course a consequence of drug abuse and excessive alcohol intake.

Food additives are in almost everything you can buy from a supermarket. Some are there to preserve the food, others to change its colour. Most of them are synthetic compounds, some with known negative health effects, and no one knows their long-term consequences.

Fresh air is no longer fresh; even in the country we cannot escape pollution from pesticides sprayed on crops. Indoors, we inhale toxic fumes from sprays and cleaning fluids, formaldehyde from insulation and carpets and, more often than we are probably aware, traces of carbon monoxide from slightly leaking gas appliances.

Free radicals are a type of pollution which it is impossible to avoid. They are produced in any process of combustion, so they enter our bodies from cigarette smoke and exhaust fumes (whether from diesel or leaded or lead-free petrol), from fried, barbecued or toasted food, from rancid or over-heated oils—and they are even produced in our bodies by the process of making energy! Yet free radicals are probably the greatest cause of illness, playing a major role in cancer, heart disease, allergy and the ageing process.

The good news is that free radicals can be disarmed. Suitable nutrients known as antioxidants, including Vitamins A, C and E, and the minerals zinc, copper, iron, manganese and selenium, can protect you by stopping the damage being caused to your body's cells by dangerous free radicals. Once again, nutrition wins the day!

Of course, the most important thing you can do is to be aware of what is actually in the food you buy and the water you drink and do whatever you can to reduce the toxic load on your body. Long-term exposure to any type of toxins will almost certainly lead to an over-worked and exhausted phase II of the liver's detoxification process, with resultant ill health.

We have managed to turn God's world into a highly toxic and dangerous place to live, but God's love and mercy have not changed and now he is giving us knowledge so that we may overcome and still live healthy and useful lives. Our loving Father shows us how the tables can be turned in our health if we will learn to do what is best for our bodies by eating the food which he created for us instead of being tempted to buy chemical-laden rubbish to put into our temples.

I hope you agree with me that we need to repent on behalf of this generation for what we have done to God's creation, both in the world around us and in our own bodies, and that then we should determine to make ourselves the best that we can be, to the praise and glory of God. The choice is ours. And praise God that when Jesus makes us clean, he does it in every sense of the word!

Wise Words

'You are already clean because of the word I have spoken to you. Remain in me, and I will remain in you'
(John 15:3–4).

For Action

- **Empty your bowels regularly!** To help achieve this, take plenty of Vitamin C—up to bowel tolerance levels; in other words, until you have a slightly loose motion every day.
- **Drink plenty of filtered or purified water.**
- **Drink plenty of dandelion 'coffee'** to stimulate the production of bile to carry toxins out of the liver.
- **Eat a healthy diet (see Appendix M),** with as much organic produce as possible, and determine to avoid all junk foods.
- **Take a multivitamin/mineral supplement** containing good levels of antioxidants and other important nutrients to protect you against the polluted atmosphere. These include Vitamins A, C and E and the minerals selenium, calcium, magnesium and zinc.
- If you suspect a build-up of toxins due to long-term medication or a history of drug or alcohol abuse, or even due to candida, **do all the above and also take capsules of silymarin** (milk thistle), a herb with renowned liver-supporting properties.
- If you suspect that the problem is deeper and requires a

nutritional approach to stimulate phase II of the liver's detox-ification processes, you need to **consult a nutritionist.**

- **As you repent to God of humankind's sin, pride and folly** which have ruined our food and our environment, and particularly of your own part in it, read again the 'Wise Words' at the end of this chapter and know that his forgive-ness cleanses you inside and out.

CHAPTER 18

STRESSES AND STRAINS— EXHAUSTED ADRENALS

'Who of you by worrying can add a single hour to his life?' (Matthew 6:27).

I quite often feel that, in Christian circles, stress is a 'dirty word'. Many of us are afraid to admit to ourselves—let alone to our friends and acquaintances—that we have any kind of a problem. We see the 'perfect' Christian as being full of joy and peace, and so we cover up the inward battles and greet our fellow church-goers with a smile which denies our inner lack of serenity. If someone approaches us with a gentle question of concern, our reply is likely to be one in which we protest too much: 'Me? Stressed? Whatever makes you think so?'

Quite apart from the scriptural exhortation to bear one another's burdens, this speaks of an unreality in our relationships which really needs to be acknowledged and dealt with if we are truly to live together as an expression of the body of Christ. In a loving and trusting fellowship, we should not only be willing to help someone else, but we should feel secure enough to expose our own weaknesses and needs, and allow others to help us.

You may possibly be thinking that stress is unavoidable,

especially in our hectic modern world, so there doesn't seem much point in saying you shouldn't have it. Perhaps you believe it is better just to put on a stiff upper lip and take it on the chin. Possibly you think that we should just get on with life and accept whatever it throws at us, pretending to others all the while that everything is fine—because as Christians, of course, we should have no areas of weakness!

'Taking it on the chin' is a figure of speech which actually indicates that stress affects us physically as well as mentally, that the problem which troubles your mind also troubles your body. Stress might give you an upset tummy, a headache, an ulcer or raised blood pressure. Even your immune system knows when you are stressed; your white blood cells, which look after you by destroying foreign invaders, know when you are angry, depressed or scared but equally they know when you are happy and relaxed, because detailed information flows along your nerves between your brain and your immune system.

So what is stress? The *Oxford English Reference Dictionary* gives several definitions, including 'pressure or tension exerted on a material object'. Another definition is 'demand on physical or mental energy', referring to what happens when pressure or tension are experienced by human beings, and the next definition is 'distress caused by this demand'. In other words, pressure or tension is one definition of the word stress, and these cause a demand on physical or mental energy which is also called stress, which in turn leads to another form of stress, which might better be labelled *dis*-tress. Stress is a little word with several facets, each one showing a slightly different angle.

To explain what causes 'pressure or tension', and how these situations make 'demands on physical or mental energy', here are some more definitions.

Pressure: the exertion of continuous force on or against a body by another in contact with it; urgency, the need to meet a deadline, etc.; affliction or difficulty; constraining influence.

Tension: the state of being stretched; mental strain or excitement; a strained state or relationship; the strained condition resulting from forces acting in opposition to each other.

I'm sure your own imagination can see how these definitions might apply in human experience.

Pressure or tension very often have an external origin, but we are also perfectly capable of producing them within ourselves, especially if we are perfectionists or live with self-made pressures and tensions due to ambition or an unwillingness to resolve a difficult relationship.

The result of pressure or tension is that we react in one or more of several different ways—with anger, fear, anxiety, frustration or even excitement. You may well be thinking that you normally experience several of these before breakfast! In fact, it is not the 'external' problems of life which are the real problem, it is our 'internal' reaction—and this is what affects our bodies as well as our minds. You just have to think how your face goes white when you have a shock, or you need to run to the lavatory if you are nervous, or you go red if you are embarrassed; it is very obvious that what goes on in your mind has a marked effect upon your body, and the most important effect is on your adrenal glands and the stress hormones which they produce.

The adrenals release three stress hormones as soon as the body has to deal with any kind of stress. They are adrenalin, cortisol and DHEA. The effect of adrenalin is to release the body's sugar stores to make extra energy available and to cause muscle tension, increased heart-rate and faster breathing. Adrenalin is produced only in the short term but cortisol and DHEA continue to play important long-term roles in enabling the body to cope with ongoing stress. In addition, they are involved in metabolism, weight control, immunity and the production of sex hormones.

When stress first occurs, the body's initial alarm reaction is to trigger the release of adrenalin. If stress continues, the adrenal glands then stimulate the release of increased amounts of cortisol but they produce less than normal amounts of DHEA. If the situation is prolonged even further, the body's resources are shunted sideways to produce more cortisol instead of DHEA, so one continues to increase while the other gets less and less.

At the same time, the hormone glands in the brain become less sensitive and unaware that cortisol levels have become too high, so they continue to send messages to the adrenal glands to produce yet more cortisol. This is the body's process of adapting to stress but it can actually learn to adapt so much that cortisol levels remain high even when external stress factors have been removed. In this situation, it becomes impossible to rest because of a feeling of 'driven-ness' to keep going and to be over-active. How many people do you know like that? Are you one of them yourself?

High cortisol also causes other problems, including the disruption of blood sugar levels and reduced ability to build protein (needed for repair work throughout the body). It also suppresses the immune system in various ways including reduced production of mucus and secretory antibodies lining the intestinal wall, which form the body's first line of defence against invading bacteria or poisonous substances. Immunity is therefore weakened.

Steroid hormones are not secreted at a constant level throughout the day, but have a rhythm of their own.

Cortisol, for instance, should be released in a cycle which is highest in the morning and lowest at night. An abnormal adrenal rhythm will have an unhealthy effect on many functions of the body, including metabolism and energy production, muscle and joint function, the strength of bones and of the immune system, the quality of sleep and the health of the skin and its ability to regenerate. Quite often, symptoms of an under-active thyroid gland such as fatigue and low body temperature are actually due to over-adapted adrenals which are producing their stress hormones in a haphazard way instead of in an orderly pattern throughout the day.

Of course, everyone has a different ability to cope with stress, depending on many different factors—inherited characteristics, diet, environmental factors, lifestyle and the length and severity of the stress itself. However, when the adrenal rhythm has been severely disrupted, sooner or later the adrenal glands become so exhausted that they are unable to produce sufficient amounts of either DHEA or cortisol. The result is chronic ill health which includes symptoms of fatigue and weakened immunity against infections and allergies.

It is usual to think of stress as a psychological problem, which of course is often the case. It can be caused by such things as emotional strain, anxiety or depression, time pressure, frustration or anger, perfectionism, having to do too many things at once and feeling out of control or unfulfilled. However, stress is also caused by lifestyle and environmental factors including pollution, shift work, extreme heat or cold, trauma or accident and even allergies. Even problems within the body itself cause stress. These include blood sugar imbalances (diabetes or hypoglycaemia), lack of sleep, poor diet, too little or even too much exercise, long-term infections and chronic pain or inflammation as in arthritis. Since these situations increase stress and stress leads to even more health problems, it is clear that the vicious circle needs to be broken.

Many nutritionists make use of a helpful diagnostic test using saliva specimens. The laboratory reports on levels of cortisol and DHEA collected at different times throughout the day, showing how their behaviour varies from the normal cycle. Sometimes the graph shows a yo-yo effect, with cortisol being high when it should be low, or low when it should be high—or staying too high or too low all through the day. A nutritionist is able to recommend a supplement programme which will help to regulate the daily cycle and nudge it gently back into a normal pattern.

Cortisol which is too high at any time of day leads to energy slumps and depression, and cortisol which is too high at midnight leads to insomnia or sleep disruptions and often causes depression and 'problems of psychological recovery', when you find it extremely difficult to get over any type of shock or emotional upset.

The laboratory report indicates how far down the slippery slope your adrenal function has fallen in its role of coping with stress, starting with partial adaptation then maladaptation leading on to adrenal fatigue and, finally, to adrenal exhaustion where the glands are no longer able to produce any stress hormones at all so that the body is totally inadequate at dealing with any type of stress, whether it be external or internal pressures or tension or illness.

Part of the problem is that, although the adrenal glands are superbly efficient at enabling us to cope with stress for considerable periods of time by varying the output of cortisol and DHEA, they are not quite so clever at reverting to normal once the stress situation is over. They remain over-adapted, leading to all the problems associated with adrenal fatigue, and there may be a sense of driven-ness or of inability to relax and unwind; the body-clock goes haywire leading to disturbed nights and unrefreshing sleep but fatigue during the day, and there may be depression or weakened immunity allowing an increase in infections or allergies—yet everything else in life is now going smoothly!

Unless something radical is done to provide the adrenal glands with the nutrients they so urgently require, there is little hope of recovery. However, nutritional therapy really can help to reverse the process which has occurred in over-adapted adrenals.

It goes without saying that every possible step should be taken to deal with the root cause of stress, both practically and spiritually. Have you discovered yet that when we can't come up with an answer ourselves, our heavenly Father says, 'Now perhaps you'll let me in on the situation?' 'Jesus looked at them and said, "With man this is impossible, but with God all things are possible"' (Matthew 19:26). Really believing these words is a good place to start.

We can also learn to co-operate with God for the healing of our minds and bodies by giving some thought to the fuel we put into the machinery—our daily food. For instance, the first practical thing we can do to help our adrenal glands is to cut stimulants out of our diet. These are sugar, salt, cigarettes, alcohol, cola, chocolate, tea and coffee. As the adrenals become increasingly exhausted, they need more and more stimulation to keep them working, so we experience cravings and addictions for any of these foods or drinks, but giving in to the cravings will only make things worse.

We need to aim for the right balance in the food we eat, having roughly twice as much complex carbohydrate (whole grains, vegetables and fruit) as protein (chicken, fish, cottage cheese, eggs, beans, lentils, yoghurt, tofu) at every meal and every snack. In fact, most people eat far more carbohydrate than protein. This control over the proportions of food we eat helps to support the adrenal glands, strengthen immunity, control blood sugar—and is also the best way of encouraging the body to burn off its excess fat.

Vitamins and minerals help. The adrenals need good levels of Vitamins C and B5, in particular. When stress has been severe and prolonged, individual nutritional help is needed to reverse its ravages and overcome resulting health problems, but you can do quite a lot to help yourself by avoiding stimulants, watching the proportions of food you eat and taking appropriate vitamins.

Exercise is highly beneficial. In situations of anger or frustration, the most we usually do is drum our fingers or make a rude remark—not enough activity to burn up the extra sugar which has been triggered by adrenalin to enter into the bloodstream! A brisk walk at the time is best, but regular exercise is a golden rule. When faced with sudden stress, simple relaxation techniques can help the body's systems get back to normal. Whoever first said, 'Take a deep breath and count to ten' knew a thing or two, but don't forget to find a daily time for resting in God's presence and drawing from him the resources which you need. In fact, the greater your need, the more important it is to make time with God throughout your day.

There was a time in my life when I was in a severe, prolonged anxiety state. I had three small children and a loving husband—but appalling ill health which had dogged me continuously for most of my life and led to extreme anxiety. The stress of it all was dreadful. Earlier in this book you have read how God set me free—partly by ensuring that I should hear him speak into my life about spiritual warfare and my need of the Holy Spirit, and partly by teaching me to take appropriate steps to improve the quality of fuel going into my machinery.

It is a combination which for me brought greater healing and wholeness than I had ever known. The combination is an expectation of God's spiritual intervention with a willingness to co-operate with him for our health and healing by taking personal responsibility—for lifestyle, for exercise and for the food we put into our bodies.

Do you believe the Bible when it says that your body is a temple of the Holy Spirit? And would you want to bring into that temple the sort of offerings which would defile it and lead to its downfall?

I learned the hard way—and it is a lesson with which I cannot argue because of the extraordinary difference it has made to my physical body and therefore to my life—that doughnuts are not an acceptable offering to bring to a holy temple!

I hope that, when you have read the final chapter, you will agree.

Wise Words
'*Cast all your anxiety on him because he cares for you*'
(1 Peter 5:7).

For Action
- **Pray about your problem,** then make a determined effort to stop worrying. There is no point in giving your problem to God and still holding on to it.
- **Allow God to speak to you and reassure you of his love** through Bible-based books such as *Listen and Live* or *My Dear Child* by Colin Urquhart (Hodder & Stoughton).
- **Make a determined effort to cut down on stimulants,**

eg tea, coffee, chocolate. Try Rooibosch tea, Barleycup, herb teas—there's plenty of choice. **Determine also to lose your sweet tooth** by cutting out all sugar and artificial sweeteners; you will feel so much better for it.

- **Eat a healthy diet** (Appendix M) and pay attention to your blood sugar levels (Appendix A).
- **Eat the right proportion of carbohydrate to protein (2:1)** by having one portion of fish or chicken with the same amount of vegetables and the same amount of wholewheat pasta, for instance, or beans with rice and vegetables, or an egg with two slices of wholewheat bread or crispbread. Don't have fruit on its own; it's mainly carbohydrate! Have it with some cottage cheese or nuts or seeds or yoghurt.
- **Keep animal fat to a minimum but make sure that you have good quality oils** from nuts, seeds and oily fish. It's good to have a daily salad with an oil and lemon dressing.
- **Take plenty of Vitamin C.** Requirements for Vitamin C vary from person to person and also from day to day, and can only be assessed by how your tummy responds to it! A helpful intake is probably between 1,000mg and 3,000mg daily, but this will be determined by your 'bowel tolerance', or how soon you experience diarrhoea.
- **Take Vitamin B5** (Calcium Pantothenate) to help support your adrenals. It works best when taken with other B vitamins, so find a good multivitamin supplement which contains these and other basic nutrients. At least 25mg of Vitamin B5 is helpful, but it may quite safely be taken up to 300mg.
- **Take Siberian Ginseng if you are suffering from long-term stress,** up to 1,000mg daily. Take it in the morning and have regular breaks (eg two months on and two weeks off). It helps the adrenals to adapt to stress.
- **If you suffer from energy slumps, depression or insomnia, or feel 'driven' and unable to 'switch off',** ask

your nutritionist to organise an adrenal stress hormone test with saliva specimens in order to be able to regulate your output of cortisol and DHEA. This is particularly helpful if you have experienced long-term stress.

- **Find time to exercise** (a brisk daily walk for twenty minutes is fine if you are physically able to manage it) so that you burn up excess sugar which has been triggered by adrenalin.
- **Make time to relax and be with God. A few minutes in his presence can offset a whole day of stress!**

CHAPTER 19

NUTRITION AS GOD INTENDED—
THE CHALLENGE!

*'Don't you know that you yourselves are God's temple
and that God's Spirit lives in you? If anyone destroys
God's temple, God will destroy him; for God's temple is
sacred, and you are that temple'* (1 Corinthians
3:16–17).

Perhaps you were prompted to read this book through an
interest in nutrition, in which case you may have been surprised at some of the other things you have been reading
about.

Or maybe you have been feeling that God wants you to
take some responsibility for your own health, to be a good
'steward' of the body he has given you. Optimum nutrition
can help you to do this by correcting biochemical deficiencies and imbalances in your body and by helping you to cultivate new eating habits which will lay a good foundation for
your future health. It is therefore a way of co-operating with
God to ensure your own well-being.

The vast majority of families today are coping with illness
of one sort or another, often mysterious and unaccountable
like multiple allergies or chronic fatigue. Many turn to alternative medicine in a desperate attempt to find an answer to

their problems, only to find themselves—as I did—enmeshed in New Age therapies. Our immune systems are finding it increasingly difficult to cope under the strain of all that is being thrown at them; our bodies were not designed to run on refined grains, chemical additives and polluted water and air.

As you saw in Chapter 17, when you read about the problems of liver toxicity, it has been estimated that in one year the average person eats 12lb of food additives and a gallon of pesticides which have been absorbed by fruit and vegetables. In addition they breathe in two grams of solid pollution from the air and take in harmful substances like nitrates from the water, and artificial hormones (steroids) and antibiotics from meat and dairy produce. Added to the problems caused by all these, there are the adverse effects of an enormously high fat and sugar intake. In the year 1900 the average person ate 10lb of sugar every year; now we each eat roughly our own body weight in the same period of time, because it has been added to nearly everything we buy!

None of these problems existed when God created men and women and placed them on the earth, neither did they exist when Jesus lived as a boy and man in Galilee. They didn't even exist as recently as the nineteenth century. With increasing scientific knowledge and skill, humanity has messed up its environment and food. As a result, the health of this generation is spiralling downwards; malnutrition is not confined to underdeveloped countries, as we have tended to think, but is in fact a very real problem in the villages, towns and cities of our Western world.

God put good food on the earth for us to eat, the best grade fuel for our machinery. In the Bible, God said, 'See, I give you all the seed-bearing plants that are upon the whole earth, and all the trees with seed-bearing fruit; this shall be your food.' And 'Every living and crawling thing shall provide food for you, no less than the foliage of plants' (Genesis 1:29;9:3, *Jerusalem Bible*). However, manufacturers have stripped our food of much of its goodness and introduced many chemical additives in order to prolong its shelf-life. In addition, we no longer drink pure water or breathe pure air.

A great many health problems are now accepted as part of normal life. Many women, Christians among them, accept and expect to have monthly misery, yet it simply does not happen when their diet is improved and their nutritional status is corrected. Wives who once with monthly regularity yelled at their husbands and burst into tears at the drop of a hat become emotionally stable. But they have had to learn that the reason they felt and acted as they did was the coffee they drank to keep themselves going, or the chocolate biscuits left by their children and eaten instead of meals—in other words, their appalling eating habits. It had never occurred to them that they were simply not giving their bodies the nutrients needed to ensure that they worked efficiently and smoothly.

The industrial revolution of the nineteenth century introduced many blessings to our Western world, but it also led to catastrophe in terms of our food. New roller-mills brought white flour—and white bread—into our lives, with longer shelf-life to satisfy the manufacturers and retailers but less fibre and nutrients to keep our bodies healthy. Clever merchandising soon made white flour seem preferable to wholemeal, and it fast became the basis of our diet. At about the same time, sugar became cheaper and more easily available so manufacturers began to include it in as many products as possible because of its preservative qualities. The sweet tooth of the general public rapidly increased and so did sales of sugary foods. Britain now leads the world in its production of cakes and biscuits made with white flour and sugar.

Other inventions allowed more meat to be included in our diet than ever before, and unhealthy hydrogenated margarine began to replace butter. Both these factors have helped to increase the amount of heart disease in recent generations.

Alongside these changes in diet, our lifestyle became increasingly less active; many of us now drive to work, sit at desks all day, spend the evenings watching television, and buy our food in tins and packets instead of digging the garden to grow it. We have created a totally artificial energy-balance.

In America it is stated that 2.5 million people die every year of preventable diseases in which diet is the main cause. As previously underdeveloped countries latch on to Western habits, their populations not only continue to suffer from deficiency diseases but also, increasingly, from our Western diseases. In these areas, problems like heart disease, cancer and diabetes, once comparatively rare, are becoming increasingly common. Yet we still think of the dietary habits which cause these situations as 'normal'. If the truth be told, in the past 150 years we have moved so far away from normality that we have forgotten what it was like. A great many people are still totally ignorant, uninterested and careless of what they put into their bodies, yet these same people will insist on four-star petrol for their cars!

Our lifestyle and our eating habits are light-years removed from those which God intended. Humankind has messed up its food, its world and its health, and things are getting steadily worse. Thankfully, public awareness has begun to increase, and environmental issues form an important part of government policies. It is becoming more generally known that lead from car exhausts affects the brains of our children, causing learning and behavioural problems. Migraines are commonly accepted to be triggered by chocolate, cheese or coffee. People are beginning to suspect that they might feel better if they knew more about which foods are good for them and how to combat the effects of pollution.

The British Medical Association has announced that aluminium has been found to play a major role in Alzheimer's disease (a form of senility), but who tells the public that aluminium is entering their bodies through their indigestion remedies and their deodorants? Who makes it known that even lead-free petrol fumes are dangerous because they contain free radicals—dangerous molecules which trigger a chain reaction of damaged cells in our bodies, leading to allergies, heart disease and cancer? Who tells us that our daily white bread helps to cause an imbalance in blood sugar levels, leading to fatigue and diabetes, and that it also causes chronic constipation, leading to bowel diseases like diverticulitis?

When we do finally grasp how much damage humankind is doing to itself, how long will it take for us to realise that part of the responsibility is ours? That we are showing no more wisdom than our non-Christian neighbours in choosing the food we buy, and that we are encouraging the situation by spending our money on junk foods which do nothing to build healthy bodies and a very great deal to harm them? As Christians, do we realise that we have a responsibility in this, that we need to repent and ask God to forgive us? Do we think of asking him to show us how we can live more closely to the way he originally intended?

Perhaps you are married. If so, doesn't it concern you that

you may be feeding your husband or wife the very foods which will one day lead to a heart attack? Or, if you are a parent, that by allowing your daughter to go without breakfast and buy crisps on the way to school you are increasing her risk of becoming anorexic and infertile? Do you want to encourage your own mother to develop brittle bones by having too few foods containing magnesium, calcium and Vitamin D? And if you are a woman, do you really want to increase your own chances of a devastating menopause by allowing your nutritional status to become too poor to cope with it?

Can we really, before God, put our heads in the sand and do nothing to prevent these situations when they are in fact preventable? I believe that only when we, as Christians, realise just how much we have abused our bodies can we repent and then learn to rebuild our bodies and our lives by choosing nutrition as God intended. We will then have the physical part of that fullness of life which we have been promised. Perhaps you have already submitted your spirit and your mind to the will of God; this is your chance to submit your body, too. The apostle John, writing to his friend Gaius, said, 'Dear friend, I am praying that all is well with you and that your body is as healthy as I know your soul is' (3 John 1:2, *Living Bible*). John would never have prayed something that was not in line with God's wishes; our Father *wants* us to be healthy!

Repenting means turning right round and starting again, so if, in order to improve your health, you are advised to make some radical changes in your eating habits, this gives you an opportunity to co-operate with God by eliminating from your diet those things (like doughnuts!) which are damaging your body, and replacing them instead with healthy foods. As a result, not only will your body be able to throw off many forms of sickness but it will be able to withstand the effects of a polluted environment and so stay healthy in the years to come.

In the process, you will have the opportunity to cultivate self-discipline and also to have an answer for God to the question he might be asking you: 'Do you want to get well?' That might seem a silly question, but Jesus asked it of the man at the pool of Bethesda (John 5:6). You might say, 'Lord, you know I want to be well—but I couldn't possibly give up eating bread, or drinking tea, or eating chocolate' or whatever else it might take to restore you to health. He asks again, 'Do you want to get well?'

Maybe at some stage you have said to God, 'Lord, I give you my life. I give you everything I have—my family, my finances, my ambitions, everything!' But have you then continued to eat just whatever food you fancied, still giving in to what Paul calls 'the evil cravings of your physical nature—to gratify its desires (lusts)'? (Romans 13:14, *Amplified Bible*). Have you in fact been saying, 'Lord, I give you everything—but I'll just hang on to this bar of chocolate, this can of drink containing who knows what, this coffee—or this doughnut'?

If you recognise yourself in this, now is your opportunity to make amends by changing to a disciplined and healthy diet and co-operating with God by putting only good food into your body. If God decides that this is the way you will become completely well, then this is the way it will come about—possibly slowly, but still surely!

On the other hand, when people begin to obey what they believe God is saying to them about their eating habits and lifestyle, God will sometimes intervene and speed up the healing process in amazing ways. I know—and possibly you do, too—of miraculous healings which have happened as a result of faith and prayer ministry. That is truly wonderful, but if God decides to heal you through a longer route involving discipline and obedience, that is his prerogative because he is God. Whichever way he decides to do it, the healing when it comes is still from him.

Of course, some day we must die—but death does not have to come through sickness and pain. It should come simply because the Lord has called us home. There is a lovely verse in the book of Ecclesiasticus, which was adopted into the Greek Bible but not accepted in the Jewish scriptures. It appears now in those Bibles which contain the Apocrypha. It says: 'The fear of the Lord will gladden the heart, giving happiness and joy and long life. With him who fears the Lord it will be well at the last, and he will be blessed on the day of his death' (Ecclesiasticus 1:12–13, *Jerusalem Bible*).

That's how I believe it is meant to be, and is in fact more likely to be if we will co-operate with God for our healing and our health. It is never too late to start; let me remind you of the elderly lady in Chapter 11. Aged ninety, she determined she would do everything she could to help her ailing body. She had chronic fatigue syndrome, gout and many minor complaints including catarrhal deafness, for which she needed to use a hearing aid. After a year, aged ninety-one, she had no fatigue, no gout and no hearing aid. Not only did she do all her own shopping and cooking, but she managed a block of old people's flats!

My own story, some of which is told in this book, is a testimony to God's love and power. Like all testimonies, it is intended to bring encouragement and hope. By living through it, I learned that God not only wanted to build my faith but he also wanted to increase my willingness to obey. Each time I have taken a step of obedience, God has poured a cup of blessing into my life; but each step of the way I have needed to hear and understand what God was saying, and then be ready to act upon it.

Paul says, 'Let your behaviour change, modelled by your new mind. This is the only way to discover the will of God and know what is good, what it is that God wants, what is the perfect thing to do' (Romans 12:2, *Jerusalem Bible*).

Sometimes people say, 'But I've always eaten just whatever I liked and I am never ill!' They manage to say it with a degree of pride, as though they themselves are responsible for this phenomenon. They should certainly praise God that he is keeping them healthy and that, as yet, he has not asked them to exercise greater self-discipline. At the same time I cannot help wondering how long he will allow this situation to continue in their lives. After all, machinery is machinery, and will not be able to run indefinitely on poor-grade fuel; it might slow down, get clogged up, or grind to a sudden halt. Unexpected heart attacks or strokes can often happen simply because the body is short of magnesium—found largely in green leafy vegetables, nuts and seeds. How many people do you know who regularly eat these foods? Without magnesium, muscles (including those around the heart and arteries) go into spasm and cut off the blood supply, thus preventing oxygen from reaching the heart or the brain. Some diseases give gradual warnings; with others, there is no second chance.

I believe totally in God's ability and desire to heal, but I also believe that he would rather we lived our lives in health than keep running to him for healing. The most obvious way we can stay in health is by providing our machinery with the best possible fuel—the wholesome, delicious food which God designed for us. Aren't you glad that we don't have to drink petrol? I feel that God really blessed us by deciding to make our body's machinery run on food!

Vitamins and minerals are simply concentrated food but they are crucial for the way in which they help to correct nutritional imbalances and deficiencies which have been responsible for malfunctioning machinery. Even when well, in this day and age of adulterated food and polluted atmosphere, a few pence spent on vitamins each day is worth its weight in gold in terms of strengthening immunity alone.

By hearing what God is saying in these days of increasing pollution and undermined bodily defences, we are giving the enemy less opportunity to invade our bodies with sickness and disease. He will use whatever means he can to make us ineffective as Christian witnesses, and though God might be glorified in someone whose faith endures through pain and suffering, the sickness itself does nothing to glorify his name.

We may be prepared to stand up in spiritual warfare when the enemy attacks our minds or attempts to damage our spirits, but by looking after our bodies we are taking an offensive stand against the devil. The temptation to have a second helping of pudding or 'just one more' piece of cake or chocolate is possibly the strongest temptation that many of us ever encounter. It is no coincidence that humankind's very first sin was to eat a tempting piece of forbidden fruit. Satan knows what he is doing where man (and woman!) and food are concerned. He knows that it is much harder to fight back from a position of weakness once his planned attack has already injured our bodies; it even becomes a battle to pray when we are ill and in the grip of pain.

So let us determine to take a positive stand to thwart the enemy's attempts to turn us into ineffective, weak and ailing Christians. Illness is no witness to the world. If that's all you get for being a Christian, who wants to know? But Jesus says, 'Do you want to get well?' (John 5:6).

I believe he is sharing his heart with you in asking you this question. He is acknowledging that he is ready, willing and able to heal you, but that it is up to you to really want it. As he asks the question again, 'Do you want to get well?', all you have to do, right now, is say 'Yes'. And when he heals you, the only honourable thing to do is to co-operate with him for your ongoing health. If God heals you of lung cancer, we can assume there's a very good chance that he'd like you to give up smoking. If he heals you of diabetes, he surely won't want you to go on eating meringues. It's all a matter of being responsible.

Mac is a client of mine who recently wrote me a letter in which he made the following comments:

After struggling with illness for over a decade, I discovered that candida was a major problem. I could find no one who understood the condition or who could help me. I tried self-help, which was costly and failed, although I read the books over and over again. I was getting nowhere.

Ten months ago, I fell on my knees beside my bed and prayed to God and I said, 'I've had enough. Please will you lead me to someone who can guide me to a nutritionist who can help. Amen.' It was as simple as that and I meant it.

Two weeks later, while out shopping, I met a friend and she told me about a friend of hers who was being helped by a nutritionist, and later that day she rang me with your phone number. I contacted you the very same day.

I would like to be able to say that the first three months of the diet were easy, but they weren't! However, I knew this was the way to go, not just my way but God's way for me. You know that since then I have improved greatly and I have also learned a great deal about diet and eating habits—so much so that I will never go back to eating so irresponsibly again. I can't do it. It's just not on. As a Christian, I would be damaging my body, which is God's temple.

I was overjoyed, to say the least, to read these words in which Mac acknowledged that he had been led by God to realise how his previous eating habits had contributed to his years of ill health, and to read also of his new determination to look upon his body as God's temple and so to treat it responsibly and with respect.

So what sort of foods should we eat? Appendix M gives you a good idea of the types of foods and the balance which will help to build healthy cells and tissues throughout your body. Read through it carefully. Eating healthily does not have to be dull or boring; it is possibly the most adventurous step you have ever taken, and you will find that it can be really enjoyable. But it does take time for your taste-buds to adapt and you need to allow for this and flavour your food with plenty of herbs, onions and tomatoes to add some interest.

If you are deficient in zinc at the moment, food will taste bland and you will almost certainly crave salt to give it some flavour, but this also will change as your zinc status improves by eating plenty of zinc-rich foods, taking a good multivitamin/mineral complex and possibly an extra zinc supplement. Foods rich in zinc include whole wheat (especially its wheatgerm content) and other whole grains, sprouted grains, pumpkin and sunflower seeds, nuts, eggs, shrimps, tuna, sardines, chicken, root vegetables, corn, grape juice, olive oil, green vegetables, salad vegetables and lentils. It shouldn't be hard to get enough zinc, yet many people are severely deficient in this important mineral.

Another reason why your new healthy diet will taste bland to start with is that sugar and sweet foods, including honey, have deadened your taste-buds. However, an initial determined effort to forego sweet foods will allow your sweet tooth to die, believe it or not. After all, you were not born with it, it has just been encouraged, so it will go away if you don't continue to feed it. It will also allow your taste-buds to come alive so that you will discover a whole new world of flavour that is hiding in natural foods.

Remember that your body is a temple of the Holy Spirit, a place to bring offerings worthy of the most high God—wholesome, health-building natural foods which, the more you eat them, the more you will come to enjoy and appreciate them.

And what should you do with the junk foods you have been eating? Well, a rubbish bin may have its weaknesses and get rusty with old age, but it cannot develop heart disease or suffer from chronic fatigue, which makes a bin the perfect place to throw your doughnuts, and your chocolate biscuits and your packets of sugar, and to pour away your cola drinks and your tea and your coffee—and whatever else you have discovered from this book that might be keeping you from less than 100% full health. Do it now! Where's the bin?

Then say, 'Thank you, Jesus, for setting me free from my own foolish and harmful cravings and lusts. I repent that, in this one area of choosing food to put into my body, I have been guilty of self-gratification and have not considered what might be displeasing to you. Thank you for giving me now the desire to co-operate with you for my healing and my health. Thank you for motivating me to make a start on a new way of eating and of thinking about the food I buy. I look to you to give me the strength and ongoing motivation which I am sure I am going to need! Thank you that all my resources are in you.

Thank you for challenging me about my attitude to food and for setting me on the road to recovery and health. Amen.'

Praise the Lord, O my soul; all my inmost being, praise his holy
  name.
Praise the Lord, O my soul, and forget not all his benefits—
who forgives all your sins and heals all your diseases,
who redeems your life from the pit and crowns you with love and
  compassion,
who satisfies your desires with good things
so that your youth is renewed like the eagle's

(Psalm 103:1–5).

IMPROVING GLUCOSE TOLERANCE (OVERCOMING PROBLEMS OF LOW BLOOD SUGAR)

Glucose is one of the simplest chemical forms of sugar. All the carbohydrate (sugar and starch) we eat is broken down into glucose—the only form in which it can be absorbed by the body and turned into energy. This glucose enters the bloodstream as soon as digestion is complete. Normally, the pancreas then reacts by producing insulin, which takes the glucose out of the blood and into the cells.

What goes wrong?

If we constantly eat sugar, the pancreas is constantly stimulated. If we eat *any* carbohydrate in refined form (white sugar, sweets, chocolate, white flour) digestion is rapid, and glucose enters the blood in a violent rush. In each case, the pancreas can over-react and produce too much insulin. Blood glucose then takes a rapid, uncomfortable drop, and may end up too low for normal functioning (hypoglycaemia). If this over-stimulation happens too often, the pancreas becomes exhausted. Now, instead of too much insulin, it produces too little so that too much glucose remains in the blood (hyperglycaemia). In its most severe form, this condition becomes diabetes.

Glucose intolerance

The regulation of blood glucose is a constant balancing act. The aim is to provide energy to the cells which need it (including the brain), and to make sure that unwanted glucose is not left circulating in the blood. If this balance is lost, both physical and mental well-being are, in turn, unbalanced. Low blood glucose (hypoglycaemia) and high blood glucose (hyperglycaemia) can have similar and wide-ranging effects: irritability, aggressive outbursts, nervousness, depression, crying spells, vertigo and dizziness, fears and anxiety, confusion, forgetfulness, inability to concentrate, fatigue, insomnia, headaches, palpitations, muscle cramps, excessive sweating, digestive problems, allergies, blurred vision, lack of sex drive and thirst.

What nutrition can do

Glucose intolerance can almost certainly be corrected by following an appropriate nutritional programme. Vitamins (especially B5 and C) give important support to the adrenal glands while things get back to normal. Chromium and Vitamin B3 are important in the formation of glucose tolerance factor (GTF), a substance released by the liver which makes insulin more potent, and the minerals zinc and manganese also play a part.

What you can do to improve your glucose tolerance

• Eat small frequent meals, preferably containing good quality protein (nuts, seeds, beans, natural yoghurt, cottage cheese, tofu, egg, chicken, etc.) and complex carbohydrate (raw vegetables, lightly-steamed vegetables, wholewheat crackers, oat cakes, wholemeal pasta, rice cakes, etc.). The best ratio is one-third protein to two-thirds complex carbohydrate—at *every* meal and *every* snack!

- Take a good multivitamin/mineral complex and any additional supplements needed to ensure the following levels:

Vitamin B3	50mg
Vitamin B5	50mg
Zinc	15mg
Manganese	10mg
Chromium	200mcg

- Aim either for two slightly larger meals and three snacks per day, or five light meals.
- Always eat breakfast, with the right foods in the right proportions, as above.
- Have an appropriate snack at bed-time.
- Avoid sugar, and foods containing sugar.
- Avoid honey and malt—they are both forms of sugar.
- Avoid refined grains (white flour, white rice, cornflour, etc.) because they are digested rapidly and glucose enters the blood in a rush. Eat wholemeal wheat flour, whole rice (brown), maize meal (not cornflour), etc. Read packet labels carefully!
- Avoid fruit juice, or at least dilute it 50/50 with water. Even if no sugar has been added (check the label!), the natural fruit sugar (fructose) still increases the level of sugar in your blood.
- Avoid foods containing preservatives and chemical additives.
- Avoid pre-packaged foods; they are almost certain to

contain refined carbohydrates and various harmful chemicals.

- Avoid dried fruit; it is very high in fructose.
- Avoid citrus fruit (oranges, grapefruit). A slice of lemon in your glass of water is fine!
- Avoid saturated (animal) fat but make sure you have a small daily intake of polyunsaturated fats (from oily fish, pumpkin, sunflower and flax seeds) and mono-unsaturated fats (olives and olive oil, avocado, almonds).
- Avoid alcohol.
- Avoid tea and coffee. Decaffeinated coffee and tea are also best avoided, as they contain stimulants other than caffeine.
- Avoid chocolate and also cola drinks. They both contain stimulants as well as sugar, as does Lucozade.
- Determine to stop smoking.
- Take regular exercise. Walking briskly enough to raise your pulse rate for twenty minutes three times a week is a target which many of us can aim to achieve.
- Do all you can to avoid stress.
- Aim to eat a healthy diet. Appendix M suggests some good alternatives to those things you will now be giving up. The anti-candida diet is very helpful for regulating blood sugar because it totally avoids all sugars (see Appendix E). Diabetics do extremely well on it, but it's just as beneficial if you have hypoglycaemia.

Acknowledgements to the Institute for Optimum Nutrition, with additions by Erica White.

PULSE CHALLENGE TEST

Some people suspect that they might be reacting to certain foods, and if this is the case I suggest a pulse challenge test. First of all, you have to avoid the suspect food for at least five days, then find a time when you can sit still for a whole hour, taking with you some of the food to be tested. After sitting for five minutes, take your pulse. (This is your 'resting' pulse rate.) Then eat the food, continuing to sit still, and take your pulse again at regular intervals throughout the hour—after fifteen minutes, thirty minutes, forty-five minutes and sixty minutes. Count your pulse over a full minute each time and write it down.

If your pulse rate has changed, look for its lowest point and its highest point and calculate the overall difference. An intolerance is very often shown by a marked increase (or sometimes a decrease) in pulse rate of at least ten beats. There might also be symptoms of some type, either during the hour or later on, because after a break of five days the immune system will have forgotten how to tolerate the culprit food, and might well react to it more strongly than before.

If there is no change in pulse rate and no other reaction, you may assume that it is safe to reintroduce the food into your diet, but if there is a change of seven, eight or nine beats, this suggests that something is happening and it would probably be a good idea to eat that food only at four-day intervals, to lighten its load on your immune system and prevent the sensitivity growing more severe.

Whole families of foods should be avoided simultaneously (eg dairy produce, gluten grains, nightshade vegetables) and then tested individually at forty-eight-hour intervals. For instance, if you are testing gluten grains, avoid wheat, oats, rye and barley for five days. On day six you test wheat, on day eight you test oats, on day ten you test rye and on day twelve you test barley. Nothing else should be eaten with the food except water, eg moisten a Shredded Wheat (which is 100% whole wheat) with water for testing wheat, make porridge with oats and water for testing oats, etc. Do not reintroduce one of the foods you have tested, even if it seems to cause no problem, until you have tested all the foods in that particular family. You will not necessarily be sensitive to all the foods in one food family (although you might), but you need to avoid them all in order to gain as clear a picture as possible for each food being tested.

You can check out several foods, one after the other, in this way. Having completed the tests on one food or food family, decide on the next and avoid it for five more days then start the new set of pulse tests. The most common culprits are cow's milk and its products, gluten grains and the nightshade family (potatoes, tomatoes, peppers, aubergines). After that, if necessary, you just go on to test any foods which appear frequently in your diet. Keep a three-day food diary and notice how often each food or drink appears, then suspect those which you have written down most often and carry out a pulse test with them.

Food sensitivities or intolerances are often caused by a

'leaky gut' allowing incompletely-digested food particles to invade the bloodstream. A leaky gut may be caused by various factors but frequently it is caused by an overgrowth of the yeast *Candida albicans* (see Chapter 10). Nutritional steps may be taken to heal the intestinal lining and in this way many food sensitivities may often be overcome, but it does take time and meanwhile it is important to pinpoint and avoid the culprit foods in order to remove a load from the immune system. The healing comes a step at a time.

CANDIDA SCORE SHEET

From Erica White's *Beat Candida Cookbook* (Thorsons)

This Candida score will help you to assess the possibility or severity of yeast-related health problems.

Risk factors

1. Have you ever taken antibiotics for longer than a month or more than once in a year? If so, score 5 ☐

2. Have you had a high-sugar diet, now or in the past, even as a child? Or have you ever lived through a high level of stress? If so, score 5 ☐

3. Have you ever had a high alcohol intake, or taken drugs? If so, score 5 ☐

4. Have you ever had any steroid treatments—pills, injections, creams, inhalers? (For women, this includes the contraceptive pill or hormone therapy) If so, score 10 ☐

Points carried forward ☐

Present symptoms

Score 1 point per line if any or all of the symptoms are occasional or mild.

Score 2 points per line if any or all of the symptoms are frequent or moderately severe.

Score 3 points per line if any or all of the symptoms are really severe or disabling.

Points brought forward ☐

5. Depression, anxiety, irritability, mood swings ☐

6. Poor memory, lack of concentration, feeling spacey or unreal ☐

7. Fatigue, lethargy, feeling drained ☐

8. Indigestion, heartburn, food intolerance, bloating, intestinal gas ☐

9. Constipation, diarrhoea, irritable bowel syndrome, stomach-ache, mucus in stools ☐

10. In women: Premenstrual syndrome, period pain or irregularities, infertility, endometriosis, loss of sex drive ☐

    In men: Prostate problems, infertility, impotence, loss of sex drive ☐

11. In women: Vaginal burning, itching, discharge ☐
    In men: Irritation of groin or genitals ☐

12. Muscle aches or weakness, joint pain or stiffness ☐

13. Eczema, psoriasis, rashes, itching ☐

14. Athlete's foot, ringworm, fungal toenails ☐

15. Cravings for sweet foods, chocolate, alcohol, bread ☐

16. Sensitivity to perfume, chemical smells, petrol fumes, tobacco smoke ☐

17. Any symptoms made worse on damp days or in mouldy places ☐

18. Dizziness, loss of balance, recurrent ear infections, deafness ☐
19. Insomnia, waking unrefreshed, drowsy during the day, need for excessive sleep ☐
20. Body odour, bad breath ☐
21. Sores in mouth, sore throat ☐
22. Nasal congestion, post-nasal drip, sinusitis ☐
23. Pain or tightness in chest, wheezing or shortness of breath ☐
24. Urinary frequency, urgency, burning ☐
25. Spots in front of eyes, burning or watery eyes ☐
26. Easy bruising, chilliness, cold hands and feet ☐
27. Headache, migraine ☐
28. Numbness, burning, tingling, lack of co-ordination ☐
29. Irritation around anus ☐

Total score ☐

Total score 75–100 There is very little doubt that you have yeast infection.

Total score 50–75 You very probably have yeast infection.

Total score 25–50 You quite possibly have yeast infection.

Total score 0–25 Count yourself blessed—but watch your step!

CANDIDIASIS AND THE ANTI-CANDIDA FOUR-POINT PLAN

Candidiasis, otherwise known as yeast infection, is an infestation of the common yeast *Candida albicans*. This is found in every human being in small amounts, but under certain conditions it grows out of control and migrates from the colon to any other tissue in the body, causing many different symptoms, both physical and mental. Particular factors which encourage this to happen are the use of antibiotics and hormone treatments (not just as medications but in the animals we eat), together with a diet high in refined carbohydrates, especially sugar. The over-use of antibiotics, steroid drugs and the contraceptive pill, together with our refined, high-sugar, present-day diet, have therefore encouraged a modern epidemic of yeast-related health problems.

When candida proliferates, it changes into a fungal form which is able to break through the intestinal wall leaving it porous, and this allows both toxins and minute particles of incompletely-digested proteins to leak from the digestive tract into the bloodstream. Not only does this lead to problems of food intolerance, but it places a heavy load on the immune system, making it even weaker in its fight against candida and other invaders.

Many people suffering from ME or Post-Viral Fatigue

Syndrome are affected by candidiasis as well as other possible contributing factors; it is very possible that the ME was initiated because the immune system was already over-stretched in trying to cope with invading candida. Bringing yeast overgrowths under control takes an enormous load off the immune system, allowing it to deal more efficiently with any other invader. I have seen many ME sufferers improve in this way.

It is helpful to use a carefully designed questionnaire (see Appendix C) to assess the possibility or severity of candidiasis. This gives a score which you can aim to reduce to zero (or as close to it as the predisposing risk factors allow) by following a suitable strategy. The only method which I have found to be totally effective is the following four-point plan:

1. Starve the yeast in the colon with a strict anti-candida diet.
2. Boost the immune system by taking a tailor-made supplement programme of vitamins and minerals. The initial levels should be taken for three months before reviewing the situation when hopefully improvements in health will show that the supplement programme may be reduced, and eventually a maintenance programme will be sufficient to meet ongoing needs. You may either work out your own programme from a book such as *The Optimum Nutrition Bible* by Patrick Holford (Piatkus), or you will need to consult a nutritionist. It is very important that the supplements should meet your personal requirements.
3. After an initial month or so on the diet and supplement programme, anti-fungal supplements should be included provided you feel on a sufficiently 'even keel'. These need to be carefully monitored as 'die-off' reaction may occur

when the yeast is killed and releases its many toxins into the bloodstream. This might seem like a flare-up of old symptoms, or it might cause flu-type aches and depression, but this can be controlled if the level of supplements is carefully regulated. A good anti-fungal to start with is caprylic acid. Take x 1 daily for at least five days before increasing to x 2 and gradually building up to x 6 daily, ie x 2 with each meal. Sometimes it is necessary to increase even further or change to a higher strength, and sometimes it is helpful at this stage to change to a different type of anti-fungal product.

4. At the same time as adding Point 3, probiotic supplements should be introduced to provide beneficial bacteria which will help to redress the balance of microbes in the colon. Preferably take one which contains Lactobacillus acidophilus and Bifidobacterium and provides at least 4 billion viable micro-organisms per capsule. (NB Keep in the refrigerator!)

Once a relief from symptoms suggests that candida is under control and this is confirmed by a drop to zero in your score for present symptoms in the candida score sheet, the anti-candida diet may be relaxed (sensibly!) for a month to ensure that this will not encourage a return of symptoms. Twice in each week, introduce some yeasted wholewheat bread, some crisp fruit (apples, pears), Edam or Gouda cheese and some skimmed or semi-skimmed milk (providing you have no dairy intolerance, of course). If there is any sign at all of a flare-up of old symptoms, stop the experiment by tightening up on the diet and try again in a few weeks' time. However, if all goes well, anti-fungal supplements may be discontinued, although it is wise to stay on a maintenance programme of vitamins and minerals and it is essential to return to the strict anti-candida diet for a further year, in order to consolidate the newly-established healthy balance of bacteria which has just been achieved in the intestines. This is probably the hardest part of all, but easy if you are determined to stay well.

After the follow-up year, it should be safe to leave the anti-candida diet, but it is valuable to see the whole regime as an opportunity to learn more about how to enjoy eating healthily because this will lay the foundation for the best possible health in the years to come. Hopefully, anyone who has experienced yeast infection will never again *want* to eat sugar or junk foods!

If you have difficulty taking anti-fungal supplements or increasing the level, this is probably because your body is already in a toxic condition and cannot cope with more toxins being released by dead candida. Stay off the anti-fungals for a month or even longer and take steps to detoxify your liver (see Chapter 17 and Appendix K).

Bringing candida under control is not easy nor is it necessarily pleasant, but with commitment and perseverance, it can be done.

ANTI-CANDIDA DIET

From Erica White's *Beat Candida Cookbook* (Thorsons)

Foods to avoid ☹

☹ *Sugar*

In all its forms, and food containing sugar. This includes brown or white sugar, demerara, molasses, syrup, honey, malt, chocolate and all other forms of confectionery, icing, marzipan, ice-cream, desserts and puddings, cakes and biscuits, soft drinks including squash and all canned drinks, tinned fruit in syrup, etc. Check all tins and packets for hidden sugar, even some frozen and tinned vegetables. Types of sugar include fructose, lactose, maltose, sucrose and dextrose.

☹ *Yeast*

All food containing it or derived from it. This includes bread, food coated in breadcrumbs, Marmite, Vecon, Bovril, Bisto, Oxo, etc., citric acid, monosodium glutamate, vitamin tablets unless the label specifically states 'yeast-free', pizza bases and most makes of pitta bread. Beware of commercial wrapped bread which claims to have no added yeast if it has been made with sourdough or sprouted grains. These products have been fermented and contain their own naturally-produced yeasts.

☹ *Refined grains*

White flour, granary flour (which is white flour with malt and added whole grains), white rice, white pasta, cornflour, custard powder, cornflakes and cereals unless 'wholegrain' or 'wholemeal' is stated.

☹ *Malted products*

Some cereals (eg Weetabix), some crispbreads and oatcakes, granary bread, malted drinks like Ovaltine, Horlicks and Caro.

☹ *Anything fermented*

Alcoholic drinks including spirits, ginger beer, vinegar and foods containing vinegar (ketchups, pickles, salad cream, baked beans), soya sauce and sourdough bread.

☹ *Cow's milk*

Also most milk products, including cream and most cheeses. (See note about yoghurt and cottage cheese.)

☹ *Fresh fruit*

Raw, stewed, made into jam or juice. (Pure fruit juice is virtually 'straight' fructose and often also very high in mould.) Freshly-squeezed lemon juice is allowed in salad dressing, mineral water, etc.)

☹ *Dried fruit*

Including prunes and the fruit in muesli. NB Figs or dates are used to sweeten some health drinks (eg Caro, Bambu, Nocaff).

☹ *Nuts*

Unless freshly cracked, because of mould. Avoid peanuts completely, even in their shells (monkey nuts) because they are very high in mould. Avoid peanut butter for this reason.

☹ *Smoked or cured fish and meat*

Including ham, bacon (even unsmoked is still cured) and smoked salmon, smoked mackerel, smoked haddock.

☹ *Mushrooms*

These are a fungus, as are truffles.

☹ *Tea and coffee*

Even decaffeinated, because they still contain other stimulants. Also avoid hot chocolate.

☹ *Cola drinks and Lucozade*

They both contain caffeine, as do Beecham's powders and some painkillers (eg Anadin, Phensic, Panadol Extra).

☹ *Artificial sweeteners*

These have been found to feed candida just as effectively as sugar, and in any case they keep your sweet tooth alive.

☹ *Preservatives*

These are frequently derived from yeasts and introduce chemicals to the body. (NB Sausages, even without preservatives, are high in animal fat and refined cereal.)

☹ *Hot spices and curries*

They destroy friendly bacteria in the intestines.

Worried? You needn't be! Coming next are lots of enjoyable alternatives. Why not treat yourself to *Beat Candida*

Cookbook? It has over 300 delicious recipes, many needing very little energy to prepare.

NB Some medications encourage the growth of yeast, especially antibiotics and steroids (including creams and inhalers, the contraceptive pill and HRT). Also, rid your home of mould or damp—regularly clean around double-glazed windows. Get rid of all your house-plants—mould from the soil becomes airborne and could be keeping you ill.

Foods to enjoy ☺

☺ *Yeast-free soda bread*

Made with wholewheat flour or other grains (see recipes following). Some bakers will make a batch for your freezer.

☺ *Bread alternatives*

Rice Cakes (these may be lightly toasted), *Oat Cakes* (malt-free), *Original or Sesame Ryvita, Wholewheat crispbreads* (read labels carefully).

☺ *Pastry*

Made with wholemeal flour, oatmeal and sunflower or olive oil, in proportions of 3:2:2. Make very moist with plenty of water and dust well with flour before rolling.

☺ *Soya milk or Rice Dream*

As milk alternatives. (Different makes of soya milk have very different flavours.)

☺ *Butter*

For spreading or cooking; otherwise for cooking use extra-virgin olive oil.

☺ *Unhydrogenated margarine*

Granose have a range of different ones, Suma is fine and new-style Flora is pretty good. Read the labels to make sure you pick the right one.

☺ *Cold-pressed oils*

Sunflower, safflower, linseed, as salad dressing mixed with lemon juice, and with an egg for mayonnaise.

☺ *Natural yoghurt*

Low-fat, unflavoured. Try it for dessert or breakfast with lecithin granules or a mixture of seeds, or with a cereal like whole puffed rice. Spread it on top of wholewheat lasagne dishes before baking, or flavour with mint as a dip.

☺ *Cottage cheese*

As a spread or a filler for your jacket potato or with salad.

☺ *Breakfasts*

Home-made muesli with oatflakes and other whole grains mixed with seeds, soaked in water and eaten with soya milk, Rice Dream or natural yoghurt. Shredded Wheat with Rice Dream. Puffed oats, puffed wheat or puffed rice or Kashi (mixed whole grains) with soya milk or Rice Dream. Porridge made with water or soya milk, sprinkled with cinnamon or nutmeg and eaten with yoghurt. Egg (boiled, poached or scrambled) eaten with wholewheat soda bread or toast and butter. Rice cakes with cottage cheese. Slices of tinned pease pudding with tomato, grilled or heated in the microwave—and many more besides!

☺ *Main meals*

Try to find a butcher selling free-range chickens and 'organic' lean meat to avoid hormones and antibiotics (lamb and rabbit are less likely to be affected), but don't forget that red meat has inflammatory properties. Enjoy any type of fish, but oily fish is particularly beneficial (herrings, sardines, mackerel, salmon, tuna). Combine a cereal with a pulse for a complete vegetarian protein, eg bean and vegetable pie or crumble, rice or bulgar with chickpeas in a tomato or soya milk and herb sauce, wholewheat spaghetti with brown lentils, tomatoes and onions.

☺ *Fresh vegetables*

All types, steamed. Aim to have a plateful of *Salad*, including *Tomatoes*, every day.

☺ *Avocados*

Good filled with cottage cheese and humus, or yoghurt with tomato purée, and topped with slices of cucumber.

☺ *Lemons*

The only fruit allowed. If adding a slice to your drinks, first scrub the peel well to remove traces of mould. Use lemon juice for salad dressing, for a yoghurt sauce with casseroled chicken and for squeezing over your fish.

☺ *Seeds and freshly cracked nuts*

These make nutritious snacks. Choose seeds from sunflower, pumpkin, flax and sesame. Keep in the fridge. NB Shelled nuts have unseen mould.

☺ *Herbs*

All kinds, fresh or dried, add interesting variations in flavour to your meals.

☺ *Mild spices*

These add interest (cinnamon, coriander, cumin, turmeric, etc.), but avoid the hot ones, especially chilli.

☺ *Hot drinks*

Barleycup and any type of herb tea or fruit tea provided it has no added citric acid or malt. Rooibosch tastes closest to 'ordinary' tea. Hot tomato juice makes a nice winter warmer. Roasted dandelion root (avoid lactose) tastes good and is wonderful for detoxifying your liver.

☺ *Cold drinks*

Mineral water, still or sparkling, with added ice and lemon not only looks good but is refreshing and delicious. Chilled tomato juice is good as a 'starter', and iced fruit teas (no citric acid or malt) make a tasty alternative to fruit juice in summer. Try whisking yoghurt with sparkling mineral water and added mint or vanilla essence.

RECIPES FOR AN ANTI-CANDIDA DIET

From Erica White's *Beat Candida Cookbook* (Thorsons)

Yoghurt soda-bread

450g/1lb/3¼ cups wholewheat plain flour
2 tsp potassium (or sodium) bicarbonate
300ml/½pt/1¼ cups natural yoghurt
150ml/¼pt/¾ cup warm filtered water

This will make two small loaves or one large one. If you want to make a batch for the freezer, a 1.5kg/3lb bag of flour and a 1 litre/1¾ pint tub of yoghurt (with 6 tsp bicarbonate and ½ litre/¾ pint warm water) makes six small loaves. Preheat the oven to 400°F/200°C/Gas Mark 6. Sift the flour and mix in the raising agent, then stir in the yoghurt and warm water. Mix together well then coat the mixture with more flour and liberally flour your working surface. No kneading is necessary. If making small loaves, divide into two and make into fairly flat, oval shapes. Cut a cross on the top. Place on a floured tray and bake in preheated oven for 30 minutes, then turn oven down to 350°F/180°C/Gas Mark 4 for another 20 minutes. To test if it's ready, tap the bottom of the loaf and it should sound hollow. Leave to cool on a wire rack. Six loaves in the oven might require a little longer baking.

Seedy yoghurt soda-bread

Make the mixture as for plain yoghurt soda bread and throw in a handful of sunflower seeds and a handful of pumpkin seeds. This makes it rather like a granary loaf!

Oaty yoghurt soda-bread

Make the mixture as for plain yoghurt soda bread except that you take out 2 tablespoons of flour from the original weight and replace it with coarse oatmeal. Instead of coating the dough with flour, coat it with more oatmeal. Top with poppy seeds and you'll be amazed at how professional it looks!

Soya milk loaf

450g/1lb/3$^{1}/_{4}$ cups wholewheat flour
1 tsp potassium (or sodium) bicarbonate
2 tsp fresh lemon juice
1 tbsp extra-virgin olive oil
Soya milk to mix (*or* 2 heaped tbsp soya flour with 350ml/12fl.oz/1$^{1}/_{2}$ cups water)
Optional: poppy seeds to decorate

Preheat oven to 400°F/200°C/Gas Mark 6. Mix raising agent with flour, stir in the lemon juice, then rub in the oil. Add sufficient soya milk to make a soft dough, probably just over 300ml/$^{1}/_{2}$ pint. Coat well with flour, shape into a round, and cut a deep cross on the top. Sprinkle with poppy seeds if using. Place on baking tray and bake for 30 minutes. Cool on

a wire rack.
To microwave, place on microwave dish and cook on High for
$6^1/_2$ minutes (600w).

Bread rolls and tin loaves

Any of the bread mixtures can be used to make small rolls.
Cook for 20 minutes at 400°F/200°C/Gas Mark 6 and then
10 minutes at 350°F/180°C/Gas Mark 4. These are lovely
eaten warm with soup if your digestion is up to it!

Tin-shaped loaves are easier to slice for toast and sandwiches
than oval ones, and for these the mixture needs to be even
more moist and sticky. Put the dough into a greased 1kg/2lb
tin, or two $^1/_2$kg/1lb tins, and smooth the top with a wooden
spoon. Bake the large loaf for 20 minutes at
400°F/200°C/Gas Mark 6 followed by 30 minutes at
350°F/180°C/Gas Mark 4, and the small loaves need just
slightly less at the lower heat.
    The addition of an egg gives bread a more cake-like
texture.

Tea bread

225g/8oz/1$^1/_2$ cups plain wholewheat flour
1 tsp potassium (or sodium) bicarbonate
2 tsp fresh lemon juice
1 tbsp extra-virgin olive oil
1 free-range egg
150ml/$^1/_4$pt/$^3/_4$ cup soya milk (or rice milk)
Sesame seeds for topping

Preheat oven to 375°F/190°C/Gas Mark 5. Sift and mix the

flour and bicarbonate powder. Stir in the lemon juice and oil. Beat the egg and soya milk together and add to mixture. Mix to a stiff batter and put into a greased $^1/_2$kg/1lb loaf tin. Bake for 45 minutes. It's easy to double the mixture and make two at a time, one to freeze.

Basic carrot cake

1 free-range egg
4 tbsp unsalted butter
2 cups grated carrot
250g/8oz/1$^1/_2$ cups plain wholemeal flour
1 tsp potassium (or sodium) bicarbonate
$^1/_2$ tsp cinnamon
2 tsp fresh lemon juice
Soya milk (or rice milk) to mix

Preheat oven to 325°F/160°C/Gas Mark 3. Beat together the egg and butter then fold in the grated carrot. Sift together the dry ingredients and mix in well. Add lemon juice and soya milk or rice milk till mixture just drops off the spoon. Pour into a loaf tin which has been brushed with olive oil or melted butter and bake for 1 hour. Allow to stand a little, then turn out carefully onto a wire rack to cool.

Variations:
Nutty carrot cake
Add a few nuts, freshly cracked and chopped.
Beany carrot cake
Add 2 tbsp of any variety of cooked or canned beans.
Carrot and parsnip cake
Replace one cup of grated carrot with one cup of grated parsnip.

Wholemeal scones

225g/8oz/1$^1/_2$ cups plain wholemeal flour
1 tsp potassium (or sodium) bicarbonate
50g/2oz/$^1/_4$ cup unsalted butter
1 free-range egg (or 2 tbsp soya flour)
2 tsp fresh lemon juice
Soya milk (or rice milk) to mix.

Preheat oven to 425°F/220°C/Gas Mark 7. Sift flour and bicarbonate powder and rub in the butter. Beat the egg and mix in, then add lemon juice and sufficient soya milk to make a firm dough. Knead lightly on a floured surface and roll out to 12mm/$^1/_2$in thickness. Cut into rounds and bake on lined baking tray. Bake for 12–15 minutes. Cool on wire rack.

GUIDELINES FOR A HEALTHY HEART—AND ARTERIES

1. Avoid SIX Ss:

a) **Sugar**
b) **Salt**
c) **Stimulants**
d) **Saturated fats**
e) **Stress**
f) **Smoking**

Let's look at these more closely:

Sugar

You don't need sugar at all, yet the average Westerner eats their own body weight in sugar every year! It is hidden in almost every product you buy, even if you don't take it directly in your drinks. Start by reading labels and buying sugar-free foods—from biscuits to baked beans. Honey is not much better, so avoid this too. It is amazing how quickly you can lose your sweet tooth if you are determined; a month without anything sweet will probably find you pulling a face next time you accidentally eat some sugar. Refined grains (white flour, white rice, cornflour, etc.) quickly turn to sugar once eaten, so you should eat only wholemeal bread and bake with wholemeal flour.

Salt

If you are a 'saltoholic' you may well be zinc-deficient. A lack of zinc leads to an impaired sense of taste, which can lead to a liking for salty foods. Supplement your diet with 20mg of zinc each day for two months and then start reducing the amount of salt you use. After a month without salt, foods that used to taste bland will begin to have some flavour.

Stimulants

Sugar is a stimulant, so are coffee, tea, chocolate and cola drinks. Stimulants provide only short-term energy, and they do it by inducing a stress reaction. In this state, the body immediately stops repairing itself. The more stimulants you have in your diet, the faster you will age. Coffee is the most harmful stimulant, and even without caffeine it still contains other naturally-occurring stimulants. As an alternative try Barleycup, and instead of tea try Rooibosch or one of the many herbal or fruit teas now available. Expect a headache when you first come off stimulants as you will actually be experiencing a form of drug withdrawal, but in a few days you should start to feel better than you have for ages.

Saturated fats

It isn't possible, or necessary, to avoid saturated fat (animal fat) completely but it is certainly wise to reduce it. Grill or bake instead of frying. Have skimmed milk and low-fat cheeses only—cottage cheese, Edam and Gouda are lower in fat than most others. Don't have more than five eggs a week—they are 66% fat. Avoid junk foods; a typical burger contains the equivalent of eight pats of butter! Have more vegetarian forms of protein, using a pulse and a grain together to obtain a really top-quality protein. (For instance, beans and vegetables with a wholemeal pastry or crumble topping, brown rice with chickpeas in a tomato and onion sauce, or wholewheat spaghetti with brown lentils in a vegetable sauce.)

Stress

You may argue that stress is unavoidable and that a certain amount is good for you. Go back and read Chapter 18 again! In relation to heart disease, stress causes your blood pressure to rise by constricting blood vessels and making your heart beat faster. Notice how you react to stressful situations, and then decide what to do about it. Good nutrition will enable your body and your mind to cope in a more relaxed way, and you'll also handle stress much better if you avoid stimulants.

Smoking

Everyone knows the high risk of lung cancer which is associated with smoking—and presumably you have so far chosen to take that risk. But did you know that smoking also increases the risk of heart disease? It triggers a process of cell proliferation, starves healthy cells of oxygen, thickens the blood and raises blood pressure. In addition, it blocks the absorption of many nutrients in your food, causing nutritional deficiencies and imbalances affecting the whole of your body.

2. Keep alcohol to a minimum

One glass of wine, spirit or beer a day is unlikely to do you any harm and may arguably do some good, but many people admit to feeling very much better if they go a week without drinking alcohol. One of its biggest problems is that it is addictive.

3. Drink plenty of water every day

Between meals, preferably filtered or bottled mineral water. It also has a much better flavour than most tap water. Add a slice of lemon!

4. Eat foods that are rich in those vitamins and minerals which are particularly good for the heart and arteries

For example, carrots, tomatoes and other red-yellow vegetables and fruits provide beta carotene, a natural precursor of Vitamin A; citrus fruit and green peppers are rich in Vitamin C; green leafy vegetables, whole grains, nuts and seeds are rich in magnesium and also in Vitamin E. Cooking destroys vitamins and breaks down fibre, which is needed to carry cholesterol out of the body, so have at least one large plate of salad every day as a main meal.

5. Aim to have at least half your diet as alkaline-forming foods

All vegetables, sprouted seeds, natural unsweetened yoghurt, buckwheat and almonds. The rest can be acid-forming foods: whole grains, pulses, eggs, fish, poultry, seeds and freshly cracked nuts. (Don't keep them too long because the oil in them will go rancid and the Vitamin E content will drop. Almonds, sesame seeds and sunflower seeds are full of calcium and magnesium and are less prone to rancidity, but brazil nuts are highest in fat and are best avoided.)

6. Eat plenty of oily fish, fresh, frozen or (occasionally) canned

Tuna and salmon count as oily fish, as well as herrings, mackerel, pilchards, and sardines—but don't fry! If you had a hot fish main meal twice a week, and a cold fish salad twice a week, it would do a great deal for the condition of your blood and arteries. Oily fish and also seeds (especially flax or linseed) are rich in an essential fatty acid called EPA which thins the blood, lowers blood pressure, reduces blood fats and cholesterol and raises HDLs, the cholesterol scavenger. Eskimos eat lots of oily fish and rarely suffer from heart disease!

7. Aim to have some good quality oil every day as a salad dressing

It should be 'virgin' or 'cold pressed' and you can use sunflower, safflower, sesame or flax (linseed) oils. If you *must* fry occasionally, use only extra-virgin olive oil.

8. Use *unhydrogenated* margarine instead of butter

Make sure that the label does NOT state 'hydrogenated'. Even if it also claims to be high in polyunsaturates, the process of hydrogenation makes the oils more harmful than saturated animal fat!

9. Read every label before you buy, and avoid all artificial additives and preservatives

10. Take a balanced supplement programme every day

A good multivitamin/mineral complex providing the nutrients discussed in Chapter 12 will help to promote cardiovascular health. If you already have problems like high blood pressure or angina, it would be good to consult a nutritionist who will formulate a tailor-made programme for you.

11. Keep fit

Aerobic exercise will help to maintain the health of your cardiovascular system. It also helps to boost your metabolic rate and keep you slim, which is good in itself because being overweight puts an extra strain on your heart and arteries. Find an exercise you enjoy—brisk walking, hill walking, jogging, cycling, swimming or aerobics—and aim to do it at least three times a week for twenty minutes at a time, or better still every day. And never ride when you could walk!

DIVERTICULITIS AND CHRONIC CONSTIPATION

Diet plays a major part in the control of this condition, since it is the low-fibre diet of our generation and civilisation which causes it in the first place by creating the wrong consistency of faecal matter which is unable to be moved along by the normal muscular contractions of the intestine. The pressure created by the build-up of this material causes the colon wall to be pushed out in little pockets, and these become a natural breeding ground for unfriendly bacteria because of the putrefactive matter which collects in them. These bacteria consume a large amount of the body's natural B vitamins, which obviously sets the scene for further problems.

Basic rules for diet

- *Plenty of vegetables and fruit*—but not citrus fruits because they irritate the gastro-intestinal tract, and no fruit at all if you also suffer from candidiasis.
- *Plenty of fluid.* At least one tumbler of water three times daily between meals, preferably on an empty tummy; first thing in the morning is good. Have lots of clear soups—vegetable, chicken, etc.

- Aim for plenty of *raw salad vegetables*, but approach this cautiously at first.
- Eat *fibre* but the best sort is partly-soluble—oats or brown rice. All grains should be whole grains and not refined, but too much whole wheat might be too rough, so alternate wholewheat bread with rye bread, rice cakes, Ryvita and oatcakes.
- Try sprinkling a tablespoonful of *linseed* (the seeds, not the oil!) on your breakfast. It makes good 'roughage' and is also anti-inflammatory, but get used to it gradually.
- Eat plenty of low-fat unsweetened natural *yoghurt*; it supplies beneficial bacteria.
- Use *margarine* made of *unhydrogenated* polyunsaturated vegetable oils and aim to use cold-pressed sunflower oil as a salad dressing every day. These are anti-inflammatory.
- Eat plenty of *oily fish*; these too are anti-inflammatory.

Things to avoid

- All *animal fats* are inflammatory. Avoid milk, butter, cheese (except cottage cheese).
- *Red meat* is inflammatory. Try to keep to fish and chicken and vegetarian types of protein (see below).
- Avoid *vinegar* completely; no salad cream, baked beans, tomato sauce or pickles.
- Avoid *tea and coffee*, even decaffeinated. Try any of the herb or fruit teas (Rooibosch is popular) and Barleycup. Tea and coffee are stimulants and will not allow your intestinal lining to calm down and be healed. Expect a headache when you first come off them; you will be going through drug withdrawal for a couple of days, but you will soon start to feel very much better.
- Avoid *sugar* as much as possible, and foods containing

sugar. Read labels carefully. (Avoid *all* sugar if suffering from candidiasis). This also is a stimulant or 'stressor' to the body.

- Avoid *alcohol* for the same reasons as sugar.
- Avoid bran—surprisingly, perhaps! Although it is effective at preventing constipation, it is also rather harsh. Its scraping action often irritates an already inflamed bowel, causing the gut wall to secrete mucus to protect itself. This has the effect of making food pass too rapidly through the bowel and so reduces time needed for the absorption of nutrients. It also increases blood sugar levels and decreases the absorption of important minerals like magnesium and zinc. There are more gentle ways of introducing the necessary fibre.

Note on vegetarian proteins

A complete protein is made up by combining a pulse with a grain, so you could try bean (any type) and vegetable pie (pastry made from a mixture of wholewheat flour, oat flour and sunflower oil with plenty of water); wholewheat spaghetti or other pasta made from rice, corn or buckwheat with a sauce made of brown lentils instead of minced beef; or chickpeas or other beans in a tomato and onion sauce with mixed vegetables and an oat crumble topping. However, if you are not used to pulses, approach them cautiously at first. Rinse them well under boiling water *after* soaking and cooking, and they should not then cause unpleasant wind in your intestines. They are a much cheaper source of protein than meat.

Supplements

- You need a basic programme of vitamins and minerals

assessed to meet your individual requirements. This will help any system of the body which is under stress.

- You need supplements supplying anti-inflammatory essential fatty acids.
- You need help with digestive processes, usually supplements providing digestive enzymes and sometimes extra hydrochloric acid for your stomach.
- You may need a herbal supplement to help with constipation or irritable bowel syndrome.
- You might need help to correct the balance of bacteria in your intestines, and this might entail dealing with an overgrowth of the common yeast *Candida albicans*. This balance is very important for the health of the colon, especially when there are areas where food can be trapped and putrefy because this is what causes the real problems of inflammation and infection in diverticular disease, once the pockets have been formed.
- You need to find a nutritionist to help you!

Exercise

Regular exercise such as walking, cycling or swimming will help to tone up your abdominal muscles surrounding the colon, which in turn will help guard against constipation. Actual tummy-strengthening exercises may also be learned.

UNDERSTANDING ARTHRITIS

There are two major kinds of arthritis as well as several less common associated conditions. The most common kind is *osteoarthritis*, which is a wear-and-tear disease. *Rheumatoid arthritis* is less common, tending to affect younger people, and it seems to be associated with a faulty immune system, perhaps triggered by hereditary factors and infections, as well as diet and lifestyle. Associated disorders include inflammatory conditions like *ankylosing spondylitis*, *gout*, *polymyalgia*, *bursitis*, *tendinitis* and *tenosynovitis* and others which are not specifically characterised by inflammation— *osteoporosis*, *fused vertebrae*, *osteomalacia*. Each of these conditions will often benefit from a specific nutritional approach, but one or more of the following nutritional factors will frequently have helped to encourage the development of any type of arthritis.

Nutritional factors often involved in arthritis

1. A metabolic imbalance of calcium with other essential minerals, eg magnesium.
2. A lack of Vitamin D inhibits the take-up of calcium into the bones from the blood.

3. Red meat, dairy products or saturated animal fats create inflammatory prostaglandins (hormone-like substances) in the body.

4. Insufficient essential fatty acids in the diet lead to failure of the immune system and susceptibility to infection and inflammation.

5. Stress, alcohol or a high saturated fat intake all block the conversion of essential fatty acids into beneficial, anti-inflammatory prostaglandins.

6. The enzyme needed for the conversion of essential fatty acids into anti-inflammatory prostaglandins requires adequate levels of Vitamins B3, B6, C and Biotin together with the minerals zinc and magnesium. A deficiency of these nutrients will increase inflammation.

7. Impurities called free radicals may be found in the synovial fluid (joint oil) causing inflammation of the joint, and they need to be disarmed by nutrients called antioxidants—Vitamins A, C, E, the mineral selenium and certain amino acids. A deficiency of these nutrients in the diet will therefore encourage joint pain. Antioxidants are depleted by stress.

8. A deficiency in the body of hydrochloric acid and pancreatic enzymes leads to inefficient digestion and absorption. The body then fails to receive full benefit of the nutrients contained in the food which is eaten, leading to a worsening of the initial deficiency.

9. Food sensitivities have been shown in clinical trials to be directly linked with arthritis. In one study of 5,000 patients who avoided all foods belonging to the nightshade family (potato, tomato, aubergine, peppers) for seven years, over 70% experienced increasing relief from pain and from some disfigurement. In another study, soya bean products were found to provoke reactions

most frequently. Other foods sometimes found to be responsible are wheat, oats, eggs, chicken and yeast. In order to discover which foods, if any, might be causing problems in your body, you should first ask yourself the question, 'Which food or drinks would I find hard to give up?' The answer might give you some clues, because foods to which we are addicted (even without realising it!) are frequently those foods to which we have a 'hidden' intolerance. If you suspect that you might be reacting to certain foods, I suggest that you carry out a pulse challenge test. If there are no foods you suspect, it still might be worth working your way through the foods mentioned above, doing a pulse challenge test with each one. An intolerance is frequently shown by a significant change in pulse rate (see Appendix B).

10. Very often people who suffer from joint pain have been told they have arthritis but this does not necessarily mean that there is any structural change or disease in their joint which would show up in an X-ray; it simply means that the joint is inflamed and painful—which the patient already knew! The cause of that inflammation, in a situation where there is definitely no structural damage, might possibly be an overgrowth of the common yeast *Candida albicans*, which would respond to a specific anti-candida approach. However, even when 'genuine' arthritis exists and is confirmed by X-ray investigations showing structural change to the bone or joint, the presence of an overgrowth of candida can make the pain worse than it would otherwise be. The only complete answer to candidiasis is a nutritional approach involving a four-point plan (see Chapter 10).

DIET FOR ARTHRITIS

Foods to avoid ☹

- Red meat.
- All dairy produce (milk, cheese, butter) other than plain yoghurt.
- Fried foods.
- Animal fats (lard, suet, meat fat).
- Refined carbohydrates (white flour, white rice, cornflour, etc).
- Citrus fruit.
- Soft fruit—strawberries, raspberries, plums, grapes.
- All stimulants (coffee—including decaffeinated, tea, sugar, salt, spices, alcohol, chocolate, cola drinks).
- Soda drinks.
- Processed foods.
- Additives and preservatives.
- Vinegar.
- Pickled, smoked, preserved foods.
- Detergent—rinse dishes thoroughly.

Possibly avoid ☹

- Wheat and/or oats.
- Other possible suspect allergens, eg eggs, chicken, yeast.
- Members of the nightshade family—potato, tomato, peppers, aubergines.
- Soya bean products.

Strict diet may well be necessary for at least six weeks before you begin to see signs of improvement. Now read on for a list of foods which you can enjoy!

Foods to enjoy ☺

- As many raw salad vegetables as possible (except possibly tomatoes).
- Vegetables.
- Seeds—sprouted and unsprouted, unless you have *rheumatoid* arthritis.
- Wholewheat flour.
- Brown rice.
- Buckwheat.
- Ryvita, rye bread.
- Millet.
- Yoghurt.
- Fish, especially oily fish (herring, mackerel, etc.).
- Free-range poultry, in moderation (not the skin).
- Pulses—lentils, beans of all types, chickpeas, humous.
- Vegetable protein—pulse and cereal combinations.
- Onions, garlic.
- Non-citrus, non-berry fruits—apples, pears, peaches, bananas.
- Tofu (soya bean curd).
- Herbs and/or potassium chloride in place of salt (Lo-Salt).

- Herb teas (try Rooibosch) or fruit teas.
- Dandelion coffee or Barleycup.
- Mineral water or filtered water.
- Cold-pressed oils on salads—sunflower, safflower, linseed.
- Unhydrogenated sunflower margarine.
- Tahini (sesame seed spread).
- Extra-virgin olive oil for cooking.

A tailor-made programme of vitamin and mineral supplements is recommended to be taken alongside the diet so that your body will have the best possible chance to carry out repairs and avoid further inflammation, degeneration and loss of function.

NB The use of aspirin is counter-productive in relieving arthritic pain because, although it blocks the conversion of food to inflammatory prostaglandins, it also blocks the conversion of essential fatty acids to *anti*-inflammatory prostaglandins! In addition, painkillers known as NSAIDs (non-steroidal anti-inflammatory drugs) play havoc with the lining of the digestive tract and this may lead to an increase in food sensitivities—a problem which might already be encouraging the arthritis!

APPENDIX K

PROTECTION AGAINST POLLUTION

Toxins are in the air, soil, water and food. Pesticides and other chemical substances invade our bodies, and over the past hundred years their levels have risen sharply and could well be overloading your body's capacity to eliminate them. Many people have higher levels of lead (from traffic), aluminium (from toothpaste, indigestion tablets, deodorants and foil), mercury (from dental fillings) and cadmium (from smoke and car exhaust) in their bodies than has ever been known before.

In addition, we are under constant attack from dangerous molecules called free radicals, which are largely impossible to avoid because they are the product of any process of combustion, so we breathe them in from car exhaust (quite apart from its lead content) and smoke from fires, factory chimneys and cigarettes. Even the production of energy within our own body cells creates free radicals but our bodies are able to cope with this level of attack; it is excess levels which put a tremendous load on our immune systems. Within the diet, polyunsaturated oils are particularly prone to free radical damage when heated, so it is safer to roast or fry with extra-virgin olive oil (which is monounsaturated) than with sunflower oil. Burnt toast and crispy bits on roast potatoes are high in free radicals!

When free radical molecules attack a cell in the body they cause a chain reaction of damaged cells, so they are now widely accepted as being implicated in many types of disease, including cancer, heart disease, weakened immunity and allergy, and they also speed up the ageing process.

Fortunately we can do something to help ourselves against free radical damage to a very large extent by ensuring that we take adequate amounts of antioxidant nutrients, mainly Vitamin A (especially as natural Beta-Carotene), Vitamins C and E and the mineral selenium. However, they should be taken with their co-factor nutrients so it is best to take a good multivitamin/mineral complex or to ask your nutritionist to formulate a tailor-made programme to meet your specific requirements.

How to reduce your pollution risk

- Avoid exercising by busy roads where possible.
- Wash all fruit and vegetables.
- Remove outer leaves of vegetables.
- Wash your hands before preparing food or eating.
- Make sure small children don't chew on paint-work.
- Avoid copper or aluminium cookware.
- Wrap food in grease-proof paper rather than cling-film or aluminium foil.
- Cut down on canned foods, which may be contaminated with aluminium or lead.
- Reduce alcohol, which increases lead absorption.
- Avoid antacids which contain aluminium salts.
- Avoid refined foods, which lack toxin-fighting nutrients.
- Check if your water pipes are made of lead; in pre-1940 houses, they usually are. If so, don't use a water softener. Soft water dissolves lead more easily.

- Don't drink or cook with water from a hot tap.
- Use a water filter, or drink distilled or spring water.
- Don't smoke—and try to avoid passive smoking.
- Avoid burnt food, and cook with extra-virgin olive oil.
- Eat lots of raw salad vegetables, fruit, nuts and seeds, so ensuring that your diet is high in antioxidant nutrients.
- Take antioxidant nutrients daily in a sensible vitamin/mineral programme.

Nutrition against pollution

It isn't possible to avoid the full extent of pollution. Luckily, research is showing that there are safe and effective ways of 'detoxifying' the body through carefully balanced nutrition.

The detoxifying diet

- Calcium and phosphorus are antagonistic to lead. They are found in seeds, nuts, green leafy vegetables and milk produce.
- Alginic acid is also a lead antagonist. It is found in seaweed (provided it comes from unpolluted waters). If seaweed sounds unappetising, try Nori. This comes in dried sheets which are crisped by heating them without oil in a very hot pan for less than 10 seconds, and then used as a crunchy garnish for soups and salads.
- Pectin helps remove lead too. It is found in apple pips, bananas, citrus fruit and carrots.
- Sulphur-containing amino acids, which are found in garlic, onions and eggs, help protect against mercury, cadmium and lead.

Supplements against pollution

- Where body levels of toxins are too high, diet alone cannot supply nutritional antagonists in doses high enough to be effective. Several research projects have shown, however, that certain nutrients are very effective in supplement form. A hair mineral analysis is the most accurate way to measure the body's levels of toxic metals.

- Vitamin C is an 'all rounder' which escorts lead, cadmium and arsenic out of the body.
- Calcium is effective against lead, cadmium and aluminium.
- Zinc acts against lead and cadmium.
- Selenium helps rid the body of mercury and, to a lesser extent, of arsenic and cadmium. High mercury levels in the body might best be reduced by taking the amino acid glutathione.
- Pectin and alginic acid are also useful in supplements.
- Magnesium and Vitamin B6 are useful for detoxifying aluminium.
- The herb silymarin, available in tablet or capsule form, is helpful for supporting the liver in its detoxification processes.
- Dandelion root is another liver-detoxifer, which works by stimulating the production of bile. Roasted dandelion root makes a very pleasant drink; grind it and make it in a filter jug or coffee machine, just like 'proper' coffee!

Many of these substances work better in combination. The overall effect should help to remove toxic loads from your immune system and strengthen your body's ability to cope with infection, allergy and harmful substances in your food and your environment.

DEALING WITH STRESS

Stress places heavy demands on our nutritional resources. We all need some stimulation or we decline into apathy, but each person has an optimum stress level. You need to understand the signs of excessive stress, and its causes. Stress (which can be anger, fear, excitement or frustration) stimulates the adrenal glands, as do certain chemical substances including refined sugar, salt, cigarettes, alcohol, tea and coffee. All these things, in excess, cause the same reaction.

The stress reaction is a physical one, for the very good reason that when primitive men and women had feelings of stress, the cause was likely to be physical danger. Their body reactions prepared them to run away fast, or else to turn and fight. The adrenal glands therefore release adrenaline, which produces a 'high' almost like a drug and gears the whole body for action. Digestion shuts down. Glucose is released into the bloodstream to fuel the nerves and muscles. Breathing, heart rate and blood pressure all increase, ready to deliver oxygen to the cells in order to burn the 'fuel' (glucose) and make energy.

If this process happens too often, or stress continues long-term, adrenaline alone is unable to cope and two other stress hormones, cortisol and DHEA, are produced in increasingly erratic amounts in an attempt to help the adrenal glands to adapt. Nutrients are used up, digestion is slow and disrupted, resistance to infection declines and allergies develop. Increasing minor problems are experienced such as headaches, stiffness, skin complaints, insomnia, depression or moodiness. If nothing is done, major problems can occur such as heart disease, diabetes, arthritis and even cancer.

The adrenal glands can become exhausted from over-stimulation. So can the thyroid, which works closely with the adrenals. More and more stimulation is needed to get them working, so there may be cravings for harmful stimulants like sugar or coffee. As the systems become worn down, there may be weight gain, higher blood cholesterol, slower thinking and reduced energy.

Action against stress

- Exercise is important for people who are stressed in any way. Obviously, it is best taken at the time the stress is experienced—a brisk walk or vigorous exercise session is good first-aid for stressed-out emotions, but if that is impossible, you will still benefit from *regular* exercise. Walking for 30–40 minutes at a pace of 15–18 minutes per mile (ie approximately 4 miles per hour) has been shown to reduce high cortisol. Aerobic exercise taken three times per week for at least 20 minutes is also helpful, but you should not over-exert yourself and it is best to have guidance from a qualified trainer.

- Simple relaxation techniques also help body systems to get back to normal. Tense your muscles as hard as you can and then relax, starting with your feet and ending with your facial muscles. Or just clench your fists tightly and relax.

- Cut down on stimulants (tea, coffee, chocolate, cola, sugar, salt) and eat the right balance of foods at every meal and every snack (two parts complex carbohydrate, ie vegetables, salad, whole grains to one part protein, ie fish, chicken, pulses, eggs, natural yoghurt, cottage cheese). It is best to eat three light meals and two snacks daily. This dietary advice helps to control your blood sugar levels and give support to the adrenal glands, and it is probably the single most important thing you can do to help regulate your adrenal stress hormones.

Long-term stress control

Your real need is to counter stress at source. Try these suggestions:

- Limit your working hours to 10 hours a day, 5 days a week, at the very most.
- Keep at least $1\frac{1}{2}$ days a week completely free of routine work.
- Make sure you use this free time to cultivate a relaxing hobby, do something creative or take exercise, preferably in the fresh air.
- Try to adopt a relaxed manner. For instance, walk and talk more slowly. A useful idea is to act as if you *were* a relaxed person!
- Avoid obvious pressures, such as taking on too many commitments.
- Learn to see when a problem is somebody else's responsibility, and don't carry it alone.
- If you have an emotional or other problem which you cannot solve alone, seek advice.
- Concentrate on one task at a time, and focus all your attention on the present.

- Learn to say what is on your mind instead of suppressing it. You don't have to be aggressive—just state your point of view clearly.
- If someone says something nice to you or about you, be grateful and believe it!
- Don't be too proud to receive help or sympathy when it is offered and you need it.
- Think about all the stresses in your life and make a list of them. Set out to find a positive attitude to things which cannot be changed, but if change *is* possible, take action! Don't let things wear you down.
- Ask a nutritionist to formulate an appropriate supplement programme for you. A laboratory test can be arranged (using saliva specimens) which can show the state of your adrenal hormones and indicate the specific nutritional help you need.
- Believe that God has an answer for your problems, and has made available for you all the resources you will ever need. What's the point of praying if you just go on worrying?
- Suggested reading: Colin Urquhart, *God's Plan for Your Healing* (Hodder & Stoughton)

Acknowledgements to the Institute for Optimum Nutrition, with additions by Erica White.

GUIDELINES FOR HEALTHY EATING

1. Make sure that at least half of your diet consists of alkaline-forming foods, ie all vegetables, sprouted seeds, yoghurt (natural unsweetened), buckwheat, and freshly cracked almonds.
2. The rest of your diet should consist of acid-forming foods such as whole grains, pulses, nuts (freshly cracked), seeds, eggs, cottage cheese, fish and poultry. Avoid refined grains like white flour and white rice as these quickly turn to sugar in the blood and have been deprived of many beneficial nutrients and fibre, causing an imbalance of vitamins and minerals and encouraging constipation.
3. Eat as much raw food as possible. Cooking destroys vitamins and breaks down the fibre in food. Have a large plate of salad at least once a day.
4. The best proportion of food at *every* meal and *every* snack is *one-third* good quality protein (fish, chicken, yoghurt, cottage cheese, beans, pulses, tofu) to *two-thirds* complex carbohydrates (all vegetables, fruits and whole grains). This gives you the best energy and the most efficient metabolism by helping to regulate blood sugar, support your adrenals and strengthen immunity.

5. Avoid sugar and other foods with concentrated sweetness. Honey and maple syrup are marginally better, but too sweet for people with a candida problem or low blood sugar. Dilute fruit juice 50/50 and soak dried fruit overnight. Many recipes using dried fruit, eg fruit cakes and Christmas puddings, you will find are sweet enough without adding sugar. Read labels and avoid products with unnecessarily added sugar like canned beans, canned sweet-corn, frozen peas, tomato ketchup, etc., and be aware of all the words which simply indicate a form of sugar. These include sucrose, maltose, fructose, dextrose, lactose, glucose and syrup.

6. When using oils other than for cooking (ie for salad dressings, spreads, mayonnaise), use cold-pressed (or unrefined) sunflower, sesame, safflower or flax (linseed) oils. Do NOT use margarine which states 'hydrogenated', even if it also claims to be high in polyunsaturates. The process of hydrogenation makes the oils more harmful to the body than saturated animal fats, so look for the word 'unhydrogenated' on the tub before you buy it. The best oils produce prostaglandins which are needed for healthy hormonal function and skin health. They also reduce inflammation.

7. Avoid frying; grill or bake instead. If you do fry, use cold-pressed (unrefined or extra-virgin) olive oil or a small amount of butter (which is actually safer at very high temperatures than sunflower oil) and cook for as short a time as possible. Cold-pressed sunflower oil may be used at baking temperatures (it makes excellent pastry!) but it is damaging if used at higher temperatures.

8. Increase fish and poultry (free-range, to avoid antibiotics and hormones). Reduce red meats like beef, pork

and lamb, ham and other high-fat foods. Even lean meat is 75% fat. Among other things, they cause inflammation and so encourage aches and pains.

9. Increase vegetarian sources of protein. A complete protein is made by having a meal which combines *a grain* with *a pulse*, like spaghetti bolognese made with brown lentils in an onion and tomato sauce flavoured with herbs and eaten with wholewheat pasta (or corn pasta or rice pasta). Another idea is bean and vegetable pie, made with beans or chickpeas mixed with any type of vegetables and covered with a crumble topping or wholemeal pastry. (A good pastry mix is made with wholewheat flour, fine oatmeal and unrefined sunflower oil in proportions of 3:3:2, with plenty of water and then dusted with plenty of flour). Both examples provide a meal which combines a grain with a pulse, the best possible food combination for protein value.

10. The essential fatty acid from oily fish is good for you, producing prostaglandins (hormone-like substances) which are beneficial for the health of your heart and arteries and so can help to reduce high blood pressure. They also reduce inflammation in the body. You get the same benefits from linseed (flax seeds). Another type of essential fatty acid is found in evening primrose oil and borage and also in various seeds—pumpkin, sunflower and sesame. It helps to correct hormonal imbalances, does marvels for your skin and is also anti-inflammatory.

11. The ideal intake of water is about 2 litres daily. However, a diet which has plenty of fruit and vegetables can supply almost half of this, since these foods are 90% water. We should therefore aim at drinking 1 litre of water a day, taken as filtered or mineral water or in

diluted fruit juice or herb or fruit teas.

12. Avoid foods with added salt. Don't add salt to your cooking, and if you must add something at the table, use Lo-Salt which has more potassium than sodium. If you think your food lacks flavour without salt this probably means that your body is zinc-deficient.

13. Avoid artificial additives and preservatives, which means avoiding most processed or 'fast' foods. Also avoid artificial sweeteners; they upset the chemical balance of the body and can even cause depression. In any case, they keep your sweet tooth alive, and that is something you are better without!

14. Avoid regular consumption of tea or coffee; preferably give them up completely! Caffeine is an addictive stimulant which plays havoc with your blood sugar levels and can cause emotional problems like depression and anxiety as well as physical problems like palpitations, migraine, insomnia, irritable bowel and cystitis. It also depletes the body of important minerals. Even décaffeinated products still contain other stimulants. Barleycup is a good alternative to coffee and Rooibosch is very like ordinary tea but without the harmful stimulants. There are many herbal and fruit teas to try. Roasted dandelion root makes a very pleasant alternative to coffee and is excellent at helping to detoxify the liver. You should also avoid cola drinks and Lucozade because they contain caffeine, as do some painkillers like Anadin. Chocolate contains some of the same stimulant drugs as tea and coffee, which is why it can be so addictive!

15. On average, if you want to drink some alcohol, don't drink more than one glass of wine, spirits or beer a day—and none at all if you have candida or low blood

sugar or an intolerance to alcohol. Sparkling mineral water with ice and a slice of lemon is delicious and refreshing. Make some strong fruit tea using two teabags at a time and then chill and serve with ice to make a variety of different flavoured drinks.

16. Smoking not only causes damage to your lungs and arteries but directly interferes with the absorption of many nutrients, causing nutritional deficiencies and imbalances which give rise to other health problems.

The foregoing changes to your general eating habits will help you to obtain and absorb nutrients and revitalise your body. It will probably take a while for your taste buds to adjust but you will soon learn to enjoy the unadulterated flavours of the natural, healthy foods. In addition, you would almost certainly find health-promoting benefits from taking a programme of supplements calculated to meet your personal requirements, and for this you may need the help of a qualified nutritionist.

If you suffer from a health problem, you probably need to follow a more specific diet than the general guidelines outlined here. A nutritional programme combining dietary changes with appropriate supplements can help to boost your immune system, regulate blood sugar, balance hormones, reduce high blood pressure, alleviate aches and pains, and overcome depression and anxiety. In fact it can transform your health.

Why not opt for optimum nutrition?

REFERENCES AND RECOMMENDED READING

Anderson, Neil, and Jacobson, Michael, *The Biblical Guide to Alternative Medicine* (Regal Books, 2003).

Bennett, Dennis, *Nine o'clock in the Morning* (Kingsway, 1971). Now available as a double edition of *Nine o'clock in the Morning* and *The Holy Spirit and You* by Dennis and Rita Bennett (Kingsway, 1998).

Davis, Adelle, *Let's Get Well* (Unwin Paperbacks, 1985).

Golan, Ralph, MD, *Optimal Wellness* (Ballantine Books: New York, 1995).

Holford, Patrick, *The Optimum Nutrition Bible* (Piatkus, 1997).

Lipski, Elizabeth, *Digestive Wellness* (Keats, 1996).

Livesey, Roy, *More Understanding Alternative Medicine* (New Wine Press, 1988).

Pfeifer, Samuel, MD, *Healing At Any Price?* (Word Books, 1989).

Sears, Barry, PhD, *The Zone* (Regan Books, Harper Collins, 1995).

Stalmatski, Alexander, *Freedom from Asthma* (Kyle Cathie, 1997).

Urquhart, Colin, *God's Plan For Your Healing* (Hodder & Stoughton, 1998).

Urquhart, Colin, *Listen and Live*, (Hodder & Stoughton, 1987).

Urquhart, Colin, *My Dear Child* (Hodder & Stoughton, 1990).

White, Erica, *Beat Candida Cookbook* (Thorsons, 1999).

White, Erica, *The Beat Fatigue Handbook* (Thorsons, 2000).

White, Erica, *The Beat Fatigue Handbook* (2nd ed., White Publications, 2004).

White, Erica, *ME: Sailing Free* (White Publications, 1996).